AF878403

Human Development

Founded 1958 as 'Vita Humana' by H. Thomae (1958–1981)
Former Editors: M.L. Langeveld (1963–1974),
B.L. Neugarten (1963–1969), K.F. Riegel (1970–1977),
W. Edelstein (1982–1987), J.A. Meacham (1977–1987),
H. Sinclair (1982–1987), D. Kuhn (1988–1996),
B. Rogoff (1997–2002)

Editor

Geoffrey B. Saxe,
Berkeley, Calif.

Associate Editor

Melanie Killen,
College Park, Md.

Designated Editor

Larry Nucci,
Chicago, Ill.

Designated Associate Editor

Terezinha Nunes,
Oxford

Advisory Editors

William F. Arsenio,
Bronx, N.Y.
Marc Bornstein,
Bethesda, Md.
Anne Colby,
Menlo Park, Calif.
Michael Cole,
La Jolla, Calif.
William Damon,
Stanford, Calif.
Ileana Enesco,
Madrid
Cynthia T. Garcia Coll,
Providence, R.I.
Jacqueline J. Goodnow,
Sydney
Paul L. Harris,
Cambridge, Mass.
Charles Helwig,
Toronto
Frank C. Keil,
New Haven, Conn.
Deanna Kuhn,
New York, N.Y.
Katherine Nelson,
New York, N.Y.
Sharon Nelson-Legall,
Pittsburgh, Pa.
Willis F. Overton,
Philadelphia, Pa.
Barbara Rogoff,
Santa Cruz, Calif.
Hildy Ross,
Waterloo, Ont.
Leona Schauble,
Madison, Wisc.
Dan I. Slobin,
Berkeley, Calif.
Deborah Stipek,
Stanford, Calif.
Sidney Strauss,
Tel-Aviv
Keiko Takahashi,
Tokyo
Esther Thelen,
Bloomington, Ind.
Michael Tomasello,
Leipzig
Elliot Turiel,
Berkeley, Calif.
James Wertsch,
St. Louis, Mo.
Sheldon H. White,
Cambridge, Mass.
James Youniss,
Washington, D.C.
Carolyn Zahn-Waxler,
Bethesda, Md.

KARGER

Printed in Switzerland on acid-free paper by Reinhardt Druck, Basel

Appears bimonthly: 1 volume per year (6 issues)

Guidelines for Authors

Human Development

The Editors and Editorial Board welcome manuscripts for review that address important issues related to human development from varied disciplinary perspectives, including psychology, anthropology, education, biology, and related disciplines. Manuscripts favored are conceptual in nature, drawing upon empirical findings and observations for illustrative purposes. Observations and findings are often used to raise theoretical issues, flesh out interesting and potentially powerful ideas, and differentiate key constructs. Scholars who are considering submitting a manuscript should consult current issues of the journal for examples of style, format, and content of published papers.

Submission

Only original papers written in English are considered and should be submitted online at:

www.karger.com/hde

Should you experience problems with your submission, please contact:

humandev@uic.edu

Editorial Office 'Human Development'
Department of Educational Psychology
College of Education
University of Illinois at Chicago
1040 West Harrison Street
Chicago, IL 60607 (USA)
Tel. +1 312-996-4856
Fax +1 312-996-5651

Conditions

All manuscripts are subject to editorial review. Manuscripts are received with the explicit understanding that they are not under simultaneous consideration by any other publication. Submission of an article for publication implies the transfer of the copyright from the author to the publisher upon acceptance. Accepted papers become the permanent property of 'Human Development' and may not be reproduced by any means, in whole or in part, without the written consent of the publisher. It is the author's responsibility to obtain permission to reproduce illustrations, tables, etc. from other publications.
The journal consists of the following types of publications:

1. Papers
2. Commentaries on Papers*
3. Replies to Commentaries by Authors*
4. Essay Reviews of Books*

* by invitation only.

Arrangement

Presentation and citation of references, statistics, punctuation and abbreviations, construction of tables, selection of headings, and indentation must be in the APA style, 5th ed., as established by the American Psychological Association and adopted as our standard. It is important that authors whose first language is not English have the paper checked by a native English speaker before submission.

Title page: The first page of each paper should indicate the title, the authors' names, the institute where the work was conducted, and a short title for use as running head.

Full address on title page: The exact postal address of the corresponding author complete with postal code must be given at the bottom of the title page. Please also supply phone and fax numbers, as well as the e-mail address for the corresponding author.

Key words on title page: For indexing purposes, a list of 3–10 key words is essential.

Abstract: Each paper needs an abstract of up to 10 lines and no more than 150 words.

Footnotes: Include only when essential. Number them consecutively and type them at the foot of the appropriate page.

Tables and illustrations: Tables and illustrations (both numbered in Arabic numerals) should be prepared on separate sheets, using APA, 5th ed., format. Tables require a heading and figures a legend, also prepared on a separate sheet. For the reproduction of illustrations, only good drawings and original photographs can be accepted; negatives or photocopies cannot be used. Due to technical reasons, figures with a screen background should not be submitted. B/w half-tone and color illustrations must have a final resolution of 300 dpi after scaling, line drawings one of 800–1200 dpi.

Color illustrations: Up to 6 color illustrations per page can be integrated with the text at the special price of CHF/USD 660.00 per page. Color illustrations are reproduced at the author's expense.

References: The list of references should include only those publications which are cited in the text. References should be listed alphabetically according to the last name of the first author. Please refer to the Publication Manual of the APA for formats required for reference citations in the text and the preparation of a reference list.

Digital Object Identifier (DOI)
S. Karger Publishers supports DOIs as unique identifiers for articles. A DOI number will be printed on the title page of each article. DOIs can be useful in the future for identifying and citing articles published online without volume or issue information. More information can be found at www.doi.org.

Examples of APA Required Formats for References:
a) Papers published in periodicals: Wertsch, J.V., & Youniss, J. (1987). Contextualizing the investigator: The case of developmental psychology. *Human Development, 30, 18–31.*
b) Books: Matthews, D.E., & Farewell, V.T. (1985). *Using and understanding medical statistics.* Basel: Karger.
c) Chapters in edited books: Hatano, G., & Inagaki, K. (1989). Sharing cognition through collective comprehension activity. In L.B. Resnick, J.M. Levine, & S.D. Teasley (Eds.), *Socially shared cognition* (pp. 331–348). Washington, D.C.: American Psychological Association.

For other examples, see the current issue. For further details, consult the *Publication Manual of the American Psychological Association: 5th Edition.*

Galley Proofs

Unless indicated otherwise, galley proofs are sent to the first-named author and should be returned with the least possible delay. Alterations made in galley proofs, other than the correction of printer's errors, are charged to the author. No page proofs are supplied.

Reprints

Order forms and a price list are sent with the galley proofs. Orders submitted after the issue is printed are subject to considerably higher prices.

KARGER

Fax +41 61 306 12 34
E-Mail karger@karger.ch
www.karger.com

© 2006 S. Karger AG, Basel

The Guidelines for Authors are available at:
www.karger.com/hde_Guidelines

Human Development

General Information

Publication data: 'Human Development' is published 6 times a year. Volume 49 with 6 issues appears in 2006.

Subscription rates: Subscriptions run for a full calendar year. Prices are given per year.

Personal subscription:

Print or Online	Print/Online combined
CHF 154.25	CHF 199.25
EUR 114.25	EUR 147.25
USD 140.25	USD 181.25

postage and handling (added to print and print/online)
CHF 33.60 Europe, CHF 49.80 Overseas
EUR 24.30
USD 45.60

Institutional subscription:

Print or Online	Print/Online combined
CHF 617.00	CHF 667.00
EUR 457.00	EUR 494.00
USD 561.00	USD 606.00

postage and handling (added to print and print/online)
CHF 42.00 Europe, CHF 62.40 Overseas
EUR 30.30
USD 57.00

Airmail surcharge: CHF 42.00 / USD 38.10
Discount subscription prices: APA

Microforms: Please direct all enquiries and orders to:
University Microfilms Inc.
300 North Zeeb Road, P.O. Box 1346
Ann Arbor, MI 48106-1346 (USA)

Subscription orders: Orders can be placed at agencies, bookstores, directly with the
Publisher S. Karger AG, P.O. Box,
CH–4009 Basel (Switzerland)
or with any of the following distributors:
Deutschland: S. Karger GmbH, Postfach
D–79095 Freiburg
France: Librairie Luginbühl
36, bd de Latour-Maubourg
F–75007 Paris
Great Britain, Ireland: S. Karger AG
4 Rickett Street
London SW6 1RU, UK
USA: S. Karger Publishers, Inc.
26 West Avon Road, P.O. Box 529
Farmington, CT 06085, USA
India, Bangladesh, Sri Lanka:
Panther Publishers Private Ltd.
33, First Main
Koramangala First Block
Bangalore 560 034, India
Japan: Karger Japan, Inc.
Yushima S Bld. 3F
4-2-3, Yushima, Bunkyo-ku
Tokyo 113-0034, Japan

Change of address: Both old and new address should be sent to the subscription source.

Single issues and back volumes: Information can be obtained through the Publisher.

Advertising: Correspondence and rate requests should be addressed to the Publisher.

Bibliographic indices: This journal is regulary listed in bibliographic services, including *Current Contents*® and Index Medicus/MEDLINE.

Book Reviews: Books are accepted for review by special agreement.

Copying: This journal has been registered with the Copyright Clearance Center (CCC), as indicated by the code appearing on the first page of each article. For readers in the US, this code signals consent for copying of articles for personal or internal use, or for the personal or internal use of specific clients, provided that the stated fee is paid per copy directly to
Copyright Clearance Center Inc.
222 Rosewood Drive
Danvers, MA 01923 (USA).
A copy of the first page of the article must accompany payment. Consent does not extend to copying for general distribution, for promotion, for creating new works, or for resale. In these cases, specific written permission must be obtained from the copyright owner,
S. Karger AG, P.O. Box,
CH–4009 Basel (Switzerland).

Disk Submission

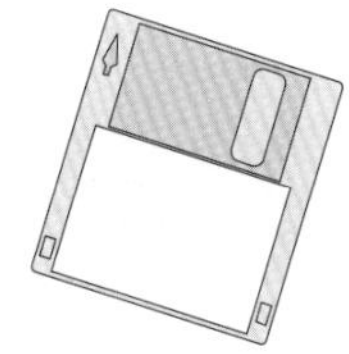

A **comprehensive version** of these guidelines for the **submission of manuscripts and illustrations on disk** can be accessed online under **www.karger.com/disksubmission** or requested as a leaflet from the editorial department.

Please follow the general rules on style and arrangement in the **'Guidelines for Authors'** of the journal. Submit a **double-spaced printout** of your manuscript matching the file on disk exactly.

Technical Information

Store only data pertinent to this manuscript. Include your fonts (screen and printer fonts for Macintosh).
For a **text only** manuscript, use a 3.5-inch disk. For **text and illustrations,** use 3.5 or 5.25 Magneto Optical Disc; CD-ROM (DOS or hybrid); iomega Zip/DOS (100 MB), or 44 MB, 88 MB or 200 MB SyQuest. Compress extensive data using ZIP format.

Data Description

Label your disk with the **title of the journal or book** for which it is submitted; a **short version** of the paper's title; your **name,** postal and e-mail address, fax and phone number; **hard- and software** used, including the version; and the **complete list of the file names.** File names consist of eight characters before the dot identifying the file and three characters after the dot identifying the application.

Text and Format

The **preferred word-processing package is MS-Word.** Other commonly used PC text programs and ASCII formats are accepted.
Update your data when you revise subsequent to the reviewer's or editor's decision and mark revisions clearly. Manuscripts accepted for publication are subject to **copy editing:** changes and/or questions will be marked in the manuscript, which will be returned to you with your disk and the galley proofs for checking.
Enter your text continuously flush left. Do not use any layout functions. Do not split words at the end of a line. **Do not use indentations.** Use a blank line before and a hard return at the end of paragraphs. **Arrange headings flush left.** Insert only **one space after punctuation marks.** Insert Greek letters, mathematical symbols etc. with your word-processing program. Use **boldface and italics** as well as sub- and superscript where appropriate. **Tables are part of the text** and should be placed at the end of the text file. Separate the individual parts of a table by lines. Use the tabulator instead of spaces. Format operation data on one line in the same column. **Legends to illustrations are part of the text** and should also be listed at the end of the text file.

Illustrations

Store illustrations as separate files: do not integrate them in your text. Export **line drawings/vector graphics** as TIF, EPS or WMF format. Use Photoshop for processing and retouching **scanned half-tone images.** Save the original scan and the processed version. Export **black and white or color images** as TIF or EPS format in their anticipated size in print.
For detailed information on how to submit illustration data on disk please consult the leaflet or **www.karger.com/disksubmission.**

KI 02 DISK

KARGER

Fax +41 61 306 12 34
E-Mail karger@karger.ch
www.karger.com

© 2006 S. Karger AG, Basel

The Journal Home Page is available at:
www.karger.com/fhde

SRCD BIENNIAL MEETING

MARCH 29—APRIL 1, 2007

BOSTON, MA

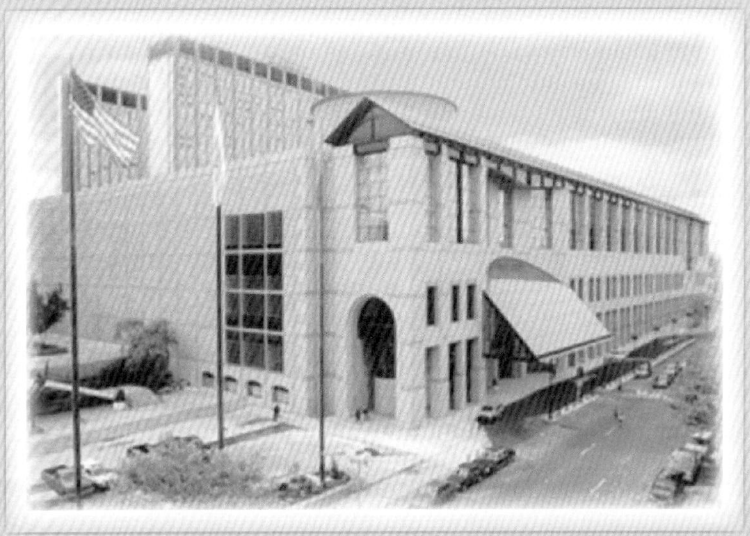

John B. Hynes Veterans Memorial Convention Center

Sheraton Boston Hotel

Register for the 2007 meeting in early October 2006.

www.srcd.org/biennial.html

Discount registration rates available to SRCD members.

Join SRCD today at www.srcd.org/membership.html

F 06578

Human
Development

How Can Research on the Brain Inform and Expand Our Thinking about Human Development?

Guest Editor
Nathan A. Fox, College Park, Md.

2 figures, 2 in color, 2006

KARGER

Basel · Freiburg · Paris · London · New York ·
Bangalore · Bangkok · Singapore · Tokyo · Sydney

S. Karger
Medical and Scientific Publishers
Basel • Freiburg • Paris • London
New York • Bangalore • Bangkok
Singapore • Tokyo • Sydney

Disclaimer
The statements, options and data contained in this publication are solely those of the individual authors and contributors and not of the publisher and the editor(s). The appearance of advertisements in the journal is not a warranty, endorsement, or approval of the products or services advertised or of their effectiveness, quality or safety. The publisher and the editor(s) disclaim responsibility for any injury to persons or property resulting from any ideas, methods, instructions or products referred to in the content or advertisements.

Drug Dosage
The authors and the publisher have exerted every effort to ensure that drug selection and dosage set forth in this text are in accord with current recommendations and practice at the time of publication. However, in view of ongoing research, changes in government regulations, and the constant flow of information relating to drug therapy and drug reactions, the reader is urged to check the package insert for each drug for any change in indications and dosage and for added warnings and precautions. This is particularly important when the recommended agent is a new and/or infrequently employed drug.

All rights reserved.
No part of this publication may be translated into other languages, reproduced or utilized in any form or by any means, electronic or mechanical, including photocopying, recording, microcopying, or by any information storage and retrieval system, without permission in writing from the publisher or, in the case of photocopying, direct payment of a specified fee to the Copyright Clearance Center (see 'General Information').

© Copyright 2006 by S. Karger AG,
P.O. Box, CH–4009 Basel (Switzerland)
Printed in Switzerland on acid-free paper by
Reinhardt Druck, Basel
ISBN-10: 3–8055–8211–0
ISBN-13: 978–3–8055–8211–7

KARGER

Fax +41 61 306 12 34
E-Mail karger@karger.ch
www.karger.com

Vol. 49, No. 5, 2006

Human
Development

Contents

KARGER

© 2006 S. Karger AG, Basel

Fax +41 61 306 12 34
E-Mail karger@karger.ch
www.karger.com

Access to full text and tables of contents, including tentative ones for forthcoming issues: www.karger.com/hde_issues

Human Development 2006;49:257–259
DOI: 10.1159/000095578

Human Development

How Can Research on the Brain Inform and Expand Our Thinking about Human Development?

Nathan A. Fox

University of Maryland, College Park, Md., USA

Although the field of cognitive neuroscience is relatively young, it has already had a significant impact on the ways we think about and measure psychological phenomena. Over the past 20 years human cognitive science has benefited from work in the more general area of behavioral neuroscience. The influence of behavioral neuroscience upon cognitive science has been multifold. Behavioral neuroscience (formerly known in some psychology departments as comparative or physiological psychology) has insisted upon the precise specification of the experimental conditions under which behavior or physiological change is observed. This includes accurate description of the stimuli that are presented and the context in which these stimuli are presented. Behavioral neuroscience has also involved a precise definition of response characteristics, leaving higher-order psychological constructs uninferred. Insistence upon specificity of stimulus and context descriptions, and reliance upon behavioral description rather than inferred psychological state have been of benefit to cognitive psychology in its attempt to understand the link between brain and behavior. Some would argue, however, that the greater influence of behavioral neuroscience has been in the areas of inquiry that include examination of what were once considered noncognitive behaviors, such as emotions and social behavior. The field of affective neuroscience links emotions, their expression and experience to the brain and brings the psychology of emotion into the realm of neuroscientific investigation [Davidson, 2000]. This influence has now spread to the area of social psychology with the advent of social neuroscience. Cognitive, affective and now social neuroscience benefit from rigorous experimental control including the accurate specification of stimuli, the context in which stimuli are presented, and the measurement of behavioral and neural change.

The focus of this special issue of *Human Development* is how these approaches can beneficially inform the developmental psychologist. Can the approaches utilized in cognitive, affective and social neuroscience and an understanding of the underlying neural mechanisms of behavior provide added value to our current approaches to understanding human development? To answer these questions, we asked three groups of neuroscientists to formulate answers for the developmental psychologist.

KARGER
Fax +41 61 306 12 34
E-Mail karger@karger.ch
www.karger.com

© 2006 S. Karger AG, Basel
0018–716X/06/0495–0257$23.50/0

Accessible online at:
www.karger.com/hde

Nathan Fox, Department of Human Development
University of Maryland, 3304 Benjamin Building
College Park, MD 20742 (USA)
Tel. +1 301 405 2816, Fax +1 301 405 2891
E-Mail fox@umd.edu

Pat Levitt and his colleague Elizabeth Hammock, systems neuroscientists at Vanderbilt University, study neural development and the influence of experience from a molecular, cellular and genetic approach. Their paper presents an overview of the ways in which work in basic developmental neuroscience informs our knowledge about the effects of early experience on behavioral development. Hammock and Levitt present examples from the areas of gene-environment interaction, and the notion of sensitive periods in development to illustrate the ways in which neurobehavioral research can be conducted. They also present two interesting approaches for understanding the underlying neural bases of social development. The first is a model system articulated by Sullivan, Wilson and Leon [1989] of early associative learning in the rodent. They have shown that odor conditioning early in postnatal life affects approach behaviors of the juvenile rat. They view this system as playing an important role in setting the physiological parameters of stress reduction as a result of the pup-mother bond.

The second approach presented by Hammock and Levitt involves the work on the neural action of oxytocin in facilitating pair bonding in prairie voles [Williams, Carter, & Insel, 1992]. The neuropeptides of oxytocin and vasopressin have been implicated in the formation of monogamous mating behavior of certain species, and researchers believe that these peptides may play a critical role in early infant-mother bonding.

At the moment, both approaches (odor associative learning and oxytocin) are framed within a behavioral system emphasizing either mother-pup attachment [e.g. Sullivan et al., 1989] or pair bonding between male and female [Williams et al., 1992]. But there is every reason to think that each may provide clues to the development of positive social behaviors and social engagement in human infants.

Charles Nelson and his colleagues Margaret Moulson and Jenny Richmond, of Harvard University, are developmental cognitive neuroscientists. They provide a compelling argument that our understanding of the development of face processing and explicit and implicit memory have benefited from an understanding of the underlying neural architecture involved in these processes and more generally from the approaches of behavioral neuroscience. Our insights into the emergence of both of these processes in the preverbal infant have benefited from the use of electrophysiological techniques, which illuminate the development of underlying neural systems. The review by Nelson and colleagues provides an excellent example of how our understanding of early brain development can aid our understanding of both normal and atypical development of face processing and memory systems.

Naomi Eisenberger, a social psychologist at UCLA who studies the neural bases of social behavior, utilizes the work done on functional imaging of the neural systems underlying 'social pain', a result of social rejection, to build a case that understanding brain systems of social behavior will inform our understanding of social relationships. In particular she links her work on brain imaging of adults during tasks eliciting social rejection to the development of an attachment relationship. Her argument is intriguing. The work on attachment formation in animals and to some extent in humans suggests that the distress behaviors of the young animal elicit attachment behaviors in adult caregivers. Eisenberger suggests that the neural underpinnings of these distress behaviors, often elicited by separation from the caregiver, may be similar to those she and her colleagues have described in adults experiencing social rejection. It may be, as she argues, that the complexity of social relationships is better understood by examining components such as the experience of social rejection or loss and linking these psychological states to brain systems in both animals and the human. Eisenberger also offers a glimpse at the issues raised by functional neuroimaging of these complex social behaviors.

There are multiple questions addressed by all of these essays and the commentary by Jerome Kagan. Does a neuroscience approach provide added value, additional important information that can assist the developmental psychologist in understanding behavioral development? Hammock and Levitt argue for a new language and approach called neurobehavioral development. They emphasize issues of sensitive periods and timing in the way in which environments affect genetic control over neural development. The focus of Nelson and colleagues on face processing and explicit and implicit memory systems provides a clear affirmative answer. Eisenberger's essay provides an interesting and innovative direction and approach for answering this question. However, the complexity of the emotional states that she studies may necessitate even further analysis before a clear answer can be provided. As Kagan argues in his commentary, complex emotional states require an explicit description of context and eliciting stimulus in order to understand the behavioral response.

Two important issues only indirectly addressed by these essays should be mentioned. First, including knowledge of the emotional quality of the stimuli or context in which cognitive processes are assessed has enriched the study of cognitive phenomena such as face processing and memory. For example, Pollak and Tolley-Schell [2003] have demonstrated that processing of face stimuli is dependent upon the experiential history of the subject. Children with a history of abuse process threatening face stimuli differently than children with no such history. Recent work on the emotional valence of words in standard memory tasks is another example of the interface of emotion and cognition.

Second, the issue of reductionism is not directly addressed in these essays. One might envision a position that would argue that all psychological phenomena can be reduced to the activity of neurons, and hence an understanding of behavior will ultimately be satisfied with only that level of explanation. In fact, as Kagan hints in his essay, even the most sophisticated of neuroimaging approaches will not capture the complexity of human psychological behavior. Our understanding of the neural activation associated with anger, distress, mistrust or hate will not help us understand the psychology of a suicide terrorist. Understanding the activity of brain systems underlying affect and cognition, and, in particular, the development of these systems and their interplay will assist but not serve as an end goal to the study of behavior.

References

Davidson, R.J. (2000). Affective style, psychopathology, and resilience: Brain mechanisms and plasticity. *American Psychologist, 55,* 1193–1124.

Pollak, S.D., & Tolley-Schell, S.A. (2003). Selective attention to facial emotion in physically abused children. *Journal of Abnormal Psychology, 112,* 323–338.

Sullivan, R.M., Wilson, D.A., & Leon, M. (1989). Norepinephrine and learning-induced plasticity in infant rat olfactory system. *Journal of Neuro*science, *9,* 3998–4006.

Williams, J.R., Carter, C.S., & Insel, T. (1992). Partner preference development in female prairie voles is facilitated by mating or the central infusion of oxytocin. *Annals of the New York Academy of Sciences, 652,* 487–489.

Paper

Human Development 2006;49:260–272
DOI: 10.1159/000095579

Human Development

How Does Neuroscience Inform the Study of Cognitive Development?

Charles A. Nelson[a, b] Margaret C. Moulson[b, c] Jenny Richmond[a, b]

[a]Harvard Medical School and [b]Developmental Medicine Center Laboratory of Cognitive Neuroscience, Boston, Mass., and [c]University of Minnesota, Minneapolis, Minn., USA

Key Words
Face perception · Fusiform gyrus · Hippocampus · Memory development · N170

Abstract
The fields of developmental psychology and developmental neuroscience have existed independently of one another for many years. This is unfortunate, as knowledge of how the brain develops can inform the study of behavioral development. In this paper, we provide two examples of how knowledge about brain development has improved our understanding of two key behavioral domains: the development of face processing and memory development. We conclude with a plea for other domains of development to integrate information from both the brain and behavioral sciences.

Copyright © 2006 S. Karger AG, Basel

Interest in the Neural Bases of Cognitive Development: Brief Historical Background

Interest in the neural bases of behavioral development is a relatively recent phenomenon that can be traced to changes in our theoretical and methodological approaches to the study of development. For example, although Piaget was trained in biology, his work was concerned with characterizing the cognitive mechanisms that underlie development, but not the neural mechanisms. Prior to Piaget, the field of cognitive development, such as it was, was dominated by behaviorism (for discussion, see Goldman-Rakic [1987]). Because of behaviorism's disdain for the nonobservable, there was virtually no curiosity about the neural bases of behavior, simply because neural activity could not be directly observed.

From the late 1970s through the end of the 20th century, neo- and non-Piagetian approaches came into favor. Despite the extensive amount of information that existed on brain development, these perspectives also favored the careful description of cognitive phenomena but not the explication of the neural processes that gave birth

KARGER

Fax +41 61 306 12 34
E-Mail karger@karger.ch
www.karger.com

© 2006 S. Karger AG, Basel

Accessible online at:
www.karger.com/hde

Charles A. Nelson
Boston Children's Hospital, Developmental Medicine
Center Laboratory of Cognitive Neuroscience
1 Autumn Street, Boston, MA 02115 (USA)
Tel. +1 617 355 0401, Fax +1 617 730 0518
E-Mail charles.nelson@childrens.harvard.edu

to such phenomena (one exception may be work by Fischer [1987], relating developmental changes in the electroencephalogram to changes in cognitive development). This all began to change towards the last quarter of the 20th century, when the ability to image the living, developing brain became possible, and when cogent arguments were made for embedding the study of behavioral development in the study of brain development [Goldman-Rakic, 1987; Nelson & Bloom, 1997]. With regard to imaging brain function, there first appeared a number of seminal studies in which the brain's electrical activity was recorded in the context of studying memory [Courchesne, Ganz, & Norcia, 1981; Hofmann, Salapatek, & Kuskowski, 1981; Nelson & Salapatek, 1986]. Within 10 years this work was complemented by the ability to image the brain's metabolic activity, using functional magnetic resonance imaging (fMRI) [Casey et al., 1995]. It was not until the mid 1990s, however, that a true neurobiological perspective began to be inserted into the study of behavioral (including cognitive) development. Here it was argued that only by understanding the neural bases of behavioral development would behavior truly be understood (for examples, see Johnson [1998], Nelson [1995], Nelson & Bloom [1997]). This perspective has become more common and accepted, although the field of developmental cognitive neuroscience is still in its infancy (for recent overviews of this field, see de Haan & Johnson [2003], Nelson & Luciana [2001]). Moreover, it has been the authors' observation that it is still not clear to many developmental psychologists why they should be interested in the brain. This is the next topic to which we direct our attention.

How Can Knowledge about Brain Development Inform the Study of Cognitive Development?

Here, and in other writings [Nelson, de Haan, & Thomas, 2006], it has been argued that our knowledge of cognitive development would benefit greatly by considering the neural bases or neural correlates of cognitive behavior. There are 3 specific reasons for making this assertion. First, the value of thinking of behavior in the context of neurobiology is that it offers a level of biological plausibility to our models of behavior. A metaphor here might be the formal proof: thus, how reasonable is it to posit the existence of a psychological construct if there is no biological evidence to support such a construct (early connectionist models come to mind in this regard)? Second, when behavioral development is viewed through the lens of neuroscience, it becomes possible to shed light on the mechanisms that underlie behavioral development, which permits us to move beyond the descriptive level to the process or mechanistic level. For example, instead of attributing the concept of infantile amnesia to the repression of early traumatic memories, we might instead attribute it to the immaturity of the neocortex, which we know is responsible for the long-term storage of memories. Finally, when one inserts the molecular biology of brain development into the equation, a more complete view of the child becomes possible – one that includes genes, brain and behavior. This, in turn, will facilitate our ability to talk at a more sophisticated level about 'gene-environment' interactions. For example, an understanding can be reached about how specific experiences influence specific neural circuits, which in turn influence the expression of particular genes, which influence how the brain functions and how the child behaves (for elaboration on all of these points, see Nelson et al. [2006]).

In the following sections we draw upon the work from two separate fields to illustrate the value added by embedding the study of cognitive development in the study of brain development.

Face Processing

The first example we will draw on pertains to the development of face processing. Scientific interest in this ability dates back at least to Darwin, who wrote about his own son's facial expressions of emotion [Darwin, 1872]. Over the past 30 years, tremendous attention has been paid to this area of research, and a consensus has emerged that to neurologically intact human adults, faces represent a 'special' class of stimuli. That is, the cognitive and neural mechanisms underlying face processing in the mature system are at least somewhat separable from those used for processing other objects (although the reasons for this dissociation are still debated [Kanwisher, 2000; Tarr & Gauthier, 2000]). Some investigators have proposed that the specialized neurocognitive mechanisms that subserve face processing reflect an innate, modular ability [Farah, 1996; Farah, Rabinowitz, Quinn, & Liu, 2000]. The logic behind this claim is that due to the adaptive value of face processing (e.g., the necessity for recognizing and discriminating among the faces of caregivers, conspecifics and predators), the neural substrates of this ability have been shaped by evolutionary history to be relatively well developed at birth, and thus require little experience in order to develop. Several lines of evidence have been taken to suggest that this may be the case.

In the normal human adult, there are dedicated regions of the brain that support face processing [Kanwisher, McDermott, & Chun, 1997]. Specifically, researchers have focused their attention on an area of the fusiform gyrus in the ventral temporal cortex (the 'fusiform face area') that is more active in response to intact faces than to a variety of other objects, including scrambled faces, houses and hands [McCarthy, Puce, Gore, & Allison, 1997; Kanwisher et al., 1997]. Damage to this region of the brain results in a condition known as prosopagnosia. Individuals who suffer from prosopagnosia are unable to recognize familiar faces despite being able to recognize familiar objects (as reviewed in Farah [1996]). Conversely, damage to other regions of the brain can sometimes result in the opposite case, in which individuals are unable to recognize familiar objects but have intact face processing abilities [Farah, 1996]. This classic double dissociation between face and object processing described in the neuropsychological literature strongly suggests that the neural substrates of face and object processing are indeed separable. Comparative studies with nonhuman primates also support the existence of dedicated neural circuitry for face processing. Specifically, single-cell recordings with monkeys have revealed that many cells in the inferotemporal cortex fire preferentially to faces compared to other objects [Desimone, 1991].

There is also some evidence that these separable neural systems are present early in development: children who have suffered damage to the ventral temporal regions of the brain early in life typically fail to develop normal face processing abilities [Farah et al., 2000]. Additionally, behavioral studies with human infants suggest that face processing represents an early-developing ability. Newborn infants will visually track moving intact faces farther than moving scrambled faces [Johnson, Dziurawiec, Ellis, & Morton, 1991] and will also look longer at schematic upright faces relative to schematic inverted faces [Mondloch et al., 1999].

Collectively, the research findings presented above have been interpreted by some to mean that the cognitive and neural mechanisms underlying face processing reflect an innate module. However, the issue then becomes how to reconcile this perspective, which has drawn primarily from adult neuroimaging and neuropsychological literature, with elegant behavioral work that demonstrates a more protracted period of face processing development [Mondloch, Geldart, Maurer, & Le Grand, 2003; for discussion, see Scott & Nelson, 2004]. Over the past few years, work in several laboratories has begun to question the view that the circuitry underlying face processing must be hard wired. The most fruitful work has viewed the problem through the lens of developmental cognitive neuroscience, and has taken advantage of neuroscientists' tools that are appropriate for use with humans – specifically, event-related potentials (ERPs) and fMRI.

ERPs represent transient changes in brain electrical activity that occur in response to the presentation of a stimulus and are recorded at the scalp. Although the spatial resolution of ERPs is relatively poor, they provide a valuable tool for investigating cognitive processes because: (1) they are entirely noninvasive, (2) the same dependent measure can be used across the entire lifespan, thereby permitting one to draw more reasonable inferences about developmental change (without regard to changes in the dependent measure), (3) their high temporal resolution (on the order of milliseconds) provides precise information regarding the timing of neural events, and (4) they do not require overt motor or linguistic responses, and therefore can be used with infants as well as with children and adults with various neurological conditions that preclude speaking or making other overt motor responses. This second advantage is especially important when evaluating claims of innateness, as in the case of face processing, because young infants can be tested using ERPs before they have had extensive experience with faces.

A large body of research with adults has revealed that faces elicit a characteristic negative deflection of the electroencephalogram approximately 170 ms after stimulus onset. This ERP component has been coined the 'N170', is observed predominantly over occipitotemporal scalp regions and is often larger over the right compared to the left hemisphere [Bentin, Allison, Puce, Perez, & McCarthy, 1996]. The N170 is of larger amplitude and shorter latency for faces as compared to other objects (e.g., houses, hands, words) and, as such, is interpreted to reflect face-specific neural processes. The N170 is also consistently of larger amplitude and longer latency for inverted as compared to upright faces, an effect that is only seen in faces and therefore considered a hallmark of face-specific processing [Itier & Taylor, 2002; Rossion et al., 1999, 2000]. Recently, developmental researchers have tested young infants using ERPs to assess both general maturational changes in the ERP response to faces [Webb, Long, & Nelson, 2005], and whether there are any components of the infant ERP that demonstrate the same functional characteristics as the adult N170. This would be expected if face processing reflects an innate, domain-specific ability.

Researchers have identified two components of the infant ERP waveform that share characteristics with the adult N170. The 'N290' and 'P400' are deflections of the infant ERP that occur over occipitotemporal scalp regions. Like the adult N170, the N290 is larger in amplitude for human faces than monkey faces at 3 and 6 months of age [de Haan, Pascalis, & Johnson, 2002; Halit, de Haan, & Johnson, 2003]. The

P400 also shows similarities to the adult N170, in that its amplitude differs for upright compared to inverted faces [de Haan et al., 2002], and its latency is shorter for faces compared to objects by 6 months of age [de Haan & Nelson, 1999]. Thus, as early as 3 months, there appears to be some functional specialization of the neural correlates of face processing, in that upright, human faces are processed differently than other objects. However, this functional specialization is not yet adult-like. Unlike the adult N170, the infant N290 does not differentiate between upright and inverted faces in amplitude or latency, a hallmark of face-specific processing. Additionally, although the infant P400 does differentiate between upright and inverted faces, this response is not specific to human faces, as it is in adults. Rather, at 6 months of age, the P400 is larger for upright than inverted faces of both monkeys and humans [de Haan et al., 2002]. It is not until 12 months of age that the infant N290 and P400 show differential responses for upright human faces as compared to all other objects, as is typical of the adult ERP response [de Haan, Johnson, & Halit, 2003; Halit et al., 2003].

Recent work has also examined the ERP correlates of face processing in children between the ages of 4 and 15 years. The ERP waveform in children resembles that of adults. However, the latency and amplitude of the N170 do not reach adult levels until adolescence, suggesting that face processing increases in speed and/or efficiency throughout childhood [Taylor, Batty, & Itier, 2004]. Additionally, the N170 response to inversion is not fully adult-like until children reach adolescence. The adult topography of the N170, consisting of a highly localized negative peak over the occipitotemporal cortex, is also not evident until mid-adolescence [Taylor et al., 2004].

The ERP studies of infants and children reviewed above elucidate the development of the neural circuitry underlying face processing and, importantly, bring evidence to bear on the debate outlined at the beginning of this section – that is, the claim that face processing abilities are subserved by an innate module that requires little experience to develop. Contrary to this claim, the evidence presented above suggests that an adult-like functional specialization of the ERP response to upright, human faces does not emerge until adolescence. The data suggest that the development of the neural circuitry underlying face processing shows a gradual specialization across development.

Developmental researchers have also employed functional neuroimaging techniques, such as fMRI and positron emission tomography (PET), to investigate the development of the neural substrates underlying face processing abilities. fMRI relies on changes in blood oxygenation to index the relative activation of different areas of the brain and thus provides a noninvasive measure of brain function that can be used with children as young as 4–5 years. PET also produces functional images of the brain by detecting changes in metabolic activity. The primary advantage of these techniques over ERPs is their high spatial resolution, which allows the precise identification of brain regions involved in various types of cognitive processing. However, neither technique is well suited for use with typically developing infants and young children: fMRI requires that participants remain still for long periods of time, while PET requires the injection of a radioactive tracer. As such, very few studies on the development of face processing have been conducted with infants and young children using these techniques.

In adults, many fMRI studies have revealed a region of ventral temporal cortex within the fusiform gyrus that seems to be dedicated to processing faces (as mentioned above). A small area of the middle fusiform gyrus, coined the 'fusiform face area', is more highly activated in response to faces as compared to many other objects (e.g., houses, cars, words, scrambled faces). This activation is typically right lateralized [Kanwisher et al., 1997]. This putative 'dedicated face processing system' in adults has been taken as evidence by some that face processing is an innate ability. Thus, developmental studies have focused on the fusiform gyrus in an attempt to evaluate whether children's functional activation of this region in response to faces is adult-like.

To date, very few studies have employed functional neuroimaging techniques to examine face processing in developing populations. In a study with 2-month-old infants, Tzourio-Mazoyer et al. [2002] found that a region of the inferior temporal gyrus that likely corresponds to the adult fusiform face area was activated more strongly to faces compared to other visual displays. Similarly, Passarotti et al. [2003] found that 10- to 12-year-old children activated the fusiform face area more strongly to intact faces than to scrambled faces. However, there seems to be developmental change in the functional specialization of this brain region. Aylward et al. [2005] found that older children (12–14 years) showed greater activation in the fusiform gyrus in response to faces compared to houses, but younger children (8–10 years) did not. Additionally, the brain activation in response to faces seems to be more distributed in infants and children than in adults. Specifically, in 2-month-olds the activation also included areas of the temporal lobe that later become involved in language processing [Tzourio-Mazoyer et al., 2002], and in older children the activation included an area in the middle temporal gyrus [Passarotti et al., 2003]. Neither of these brain regions is typically activated in response to faces in adults, suggesting that the anatomical specialization of face processing systems continues to develop into adolescence.

Thus, converging evidence from neuroimaging (i.e., fMRI, PET) and neurophysiological (e.g., ERP) studies with infants and children indicates that the basic organization of the neural circuitry subserving face processing continues to develop well into childhood and adolescence. The protracted development of the neural substrates of face processing, as evident in the gradual functional specialization of its ERP correlates and brain regions such as the fusiform gyrus, is not consistent with the claim that face processing represents an innate, domain-specific ability. As such, researchers taking a developmental cognitive neuroscience perspective have rejected claims of innateness and instead propose a new framework for understanding the development of face processing. Nelson [2001] argues that the development of face processing reflects an experience-expectant process, in which cortical specialization for face processing develops as a result of species-typical experiences occurring within a sensitive period of development.

Memory

The second example we will address concerns how neuroscience has informed the study of memory development. In the 1950s, neuropsychologists first documented a case of a patient who, as the result of a temporal lobe resection, had a profound inability to form new memories [Scoville & Milner, 1957]. While H.M. was severely impaired on tests of long-term memory that required the recall or recognition of recently learned material, performance on certain kinds of priming, conditioning and skill learning tasks remained intact [Cohen, Eichenbaum, Deacedo, & Corkin, 1985; Corkin, 1968; Scoville, 1968]. To explain this apparent dissociation between remembering 'what' and remembering 'how', researchers suggested that there may be multiple memory systems. These different memory systems have been described interchangeably as declarative or explicit memory versus nondeclarative or implicit memory [Cohen & Squire, 1980; Graf & Schacter, 1985; Squire, 1994]. Since the 1950s, studies of human amnesics and lesioned animals have provided evidence that explicit memory is dependent on the hippocampus and surrounding cortex in the medial temporal lobe (MTL), while implicit memory depends on areas of the striatum and cerebellum.

The multiple memory systems perspective sparked a debate about the nature of memory development. Some researchers suggest that while implicit memory is present from very early in life, the development of adult-like explicit memory does not occur until around 8 months of age [Nelson, 1995; Schacter & Moscovitch, 1984]. Others argue that there is no evidence for a qualitative change in the nature of infants' memory during the first year, but rather that explicit and implicit memory systems develop gradually and in parallel starting early in life [Rovee-Collier, 1997; Rovee-Collier, Hayne, & Colombo, 2001].

The evidence in favor of each side of the debate comes from very different perspectives. Those in favor of discontinuity in memory system development argue from a brain-based perspective, suggesting that the brain structures responsible for adult-like explicit memory are not functionally mature until late in infancy. For example, Nelson [1995] suggests that while the areas of the striatum and cerebellum that support implicit memory are functioning early in life, the brain systems responsible for adult-like explicit memory, including the hippocampus and surrounding cortex, do not come online until the second half of the first year of life. In contrast, evidence for continuity in memory system development comes from a behavior-based perspective. Rovee-Collier and colleagues have shown that when infants of different ages are tested on the same task across the first year of life, memory development appears to be a gradual and continuous process [Hartshorn et al., 1998; Rovee-Collier, 1997; Rovee-Collier et al., 2001].

There are problems with each of these perspectives. The brain-based approach lacks evidence from empirical studies of brain development in human infants and children. Given the difficulty of using modern neuroimaging techniques such as MRI with developing populations, researchers interested in the development of brain regions involved in explicit and implicit memory have largely been limited to making inferences from neuropsychological studies of adults [McDonough, Mandler, McKee, & Squire, 1995; McKee & Squire, 1993] and neuroanatomical studies of animals [Seress, 2001; Seress & Ribak, 1995]. Although such strategies are widely accepted, some researchers have suggested that it is inappropriate to draw analogies between brain-damaged adults and developing infants, whose brains are intact but functionally immature [Rovee-Collier, 1997]. Additionally, it is problematic to infer functional development of brain systems in human infants, from studies of the structural development of brain regions in animals [Seress, 2001].

In the case of the behavior-based approach, researchers' conclusions are limited by the fact that they must use infants' overt behavior as an index of their memory. Different tasks are typically used to measure memory in infants of different ages because of the kind of behavior that can be used to index memory changes with development. For example, while memory tasks that are used with very young infants typically involve very simple motoric responses (e.g., eye movements, foot kicks), later in the first year of life infants are able to exhibit memory using more sophisticated motor behavior (e.g., reaching, lever pressing, reproducing actions with objects). There are few tasks that are suitable for use with infants of different ages across the first year of life. As such, it is difficult for researchers to make conclusions about age-related changes in memory, independent of changes in motoric capabilities [Rovee-Collier et al., 2001].

By integrating the study of brain and behavior development, studies taking a developmental cognitive neuroscience perspective on the issue of memory development have the potential to overcome many of the difficulties described above. First, by using neuroimaging techniques to directly measure how age-related changes in the brain are related to memory development, researchers can truly evaluate conclusions that have been drawn from the adult and animal literature. Second, techniques such as ERPs may be correlated with behavior but do not require a motoric response; thus, researchers may overcome issues of developmental changes in motor abilities disguising age-related differences in memory performance.

There are a number of characteristic components of the infant ERP waveform that have proven to be of interest in the study of memory development. The Nc, a mid-latency negative component that is evident over frontocentral leads, is a robust feature of the infant ERP waveform and is thought to reflect obligatory attention. Although not considered a direct index of memory, the Nc is often modulated by stimulus novelty [Bauer, Wiebe, Carver, Waters, & Nelson, 2003; Carver, Bauer, & Nelson, 2000; de Haan & Nelson, 1997; Reynolds & Richards, 2005; Richards, 2003]. In addition, late slow-wave activity is sensitive to both the frequency and familiarity of stimulus presentation and is thought to index memory processing more directly [Nelson & Collins, 1991; Nelson & Collins, 1992].

The modified oddball paradigm has been used most often to study the ERP correlates of infant memory [Nelson & Collins, 1991; Nelson & Collins, 1992; Reynolds & Richards, 2005; Richards, 2003]. In this paradigm, infants are familiarized with two stimuli. Following familiarization, one stimulus is presented on 60% of trials (frequent familiar) and the other is presented on 20% of trials (infrequent familiar). An infrequent novel stimulus is presented on the remaining 20% of trials. Studies using this paradigm have shown that following the Nc, the infant ERP response may take one of three forms: a positive slow wave, negative slow wave or a return to baseline. The positive slow wave is thought to index memory updating of a partially encoded or forgotten stimulus. The negative slow wave is often seen in response to a novel stimulus that is presented in the context of familiar stimuli and is thought to reflect novelty detection. A return to baseline is interpreted as evidence of a fully encoded stimulus that does not require additional processing [Nelson, 1997].

There is considerable developmental change in the pattern of late slow-wave activity that is seen in response to novel and familiar stimuli. Nelson and Collins [1991] and Nelson and Collins [1992] have shown that in 4-month-olds, slow-wave activity does not differentiate between novel and familiar stimuli. In 6-month-olds, however, late components are modulated by both the familiarity and frequency of stimulus presentation. Infants fully encoded the familiar stimulus when it was presented frequently; however, the infrequent familiar stimulus required memory updating. By 8 months of age, slow-wave activity differentiated between novel and familiar stimuli irrespective of the relative frequency of stimulus presentation, indicating that even an infrequent presentation was sufficient for infants to maintain a representation of a familiar stimulus.

In summary, ERP research with human infants has yielded replicable patterns of brain activity that are related to attention and recognition memory (for an example of a longitudinal ERP study with infants concerned with these processes, see Webb et al. [2005]). The Nc, which is thought to reflect obligatory attention, is evident in the ERP waveform even in very young infants. Although the Nc is often sensitive to stimulus novelty, recent source models locating dipoles in the prefrontal and cingulate cortex are consistent with a primary role in attention [Reynolds & Richards, 2005]. Patterns of late slow-wave activity in the infant ERP waveform appear not to be modulated by memory until 6 months of age. This evidence is consistent with the view that the brain regions responsible for explicit memory 'come online' late in the first year of life. Future developments in source localization techniques will allow researchers to elucidate the neural generators of this late slow-wave activity and thus determine whether it in fact reflects the neural correlates of explicit memory in infancy.

Although the major debate over when explicit memory emerges has focused on memory in infancy, there are major developmental changes in explicit memory that continue into early and middle childhood. While the temporal resolution of ERPs continues to make electrophysiological techniques appealing in investigations of the timing of cognitive processes during childhood [Cycowicz, 2000; Cycowicz, Friedman, & Duff, 2003; Marshall, Drummey, Fox, & Newcombe, 2000], in studies of older children researchers are also able to capitalize on the spatial resolution of techniques such as fMRI.

Although 10 years have passed since the first study was published using fMRI to investigate cognitive development in children [Casey et al., 1995], there have been relatively few studies of explicit memory development. Similar to the face processing literature reviewed above, fMRI studies investigating brain activation during explicit memory tasks have shown that children and adults differ in the extent, rather than the location of brain activation. For example, Menon, Boyett-Anderson and Reiss [2005] recorded brain activity during encoding in a group of 11- to 19-year-olds and subsequently tested them for recognition. In all participants, encoding was associated with activation in areas of striate and extrastriate cortex, along with the hippocampus, entorhinal cortex and parahippocampal gyrus in the MTL. However, the extent of activation in the left MTL was greater for younger children than for older children [Menon et al., 2005]. Along with this fine-tuning of neural activation with age, Menon et al. [2005] also reported age-related increases in functional connectivity between the left entorhinal cortex and left prefrontal cortex across this age range. This result is consistent with suggestions that increasing connectivity between the MTL and areas of the frontal cortex that have a protracted period of development may at least in part account for age-related changes in memory across childhood [Nelson, 1995].

Thomas and colleagues have taken an innovative approach to understanding the neural bases of memory development by combining ERP and fMRI techniques [Hunt, Couperus, Nelson, & Thomas, 2004; Thomas et al., 2004]. In one study, 7- to 8-year-old children and adults were tested using a continuous recognition task in two sessions, once while an fMRI scan was performed and once while ERPs were recorded. The continuous recognition task requires participants to judge whether each of a series of stimuli is new or has been presented before (old), thus requiring both encoding and retrieval processes. Preliminary fMRI results indicated that adults and children activated similar areas of the MTL and inferior temporal lobe in performing the continuous recognition task; however, there were developmental differences in the extent to which the prefrontal cortex was recruited. ERP analyses showed that in both children and adults, early (300–500 ms) and late (800–1,200 ms) ERP components recorded over parietal scalp regions differentiated between old and new stimuli. Source modeling identified dipoles in the MTL that accounted for these components in both adults and children. In combination, fMRI and ERP techniques have the potential to provide complementary information about both the brain regions that are recruited in performing a memory task and the timing of cognitive processes related to task performance.

By integrating the study of brain and behavior, developmental cognitive neuroscientists have only recently begun to make significant contributions to our understanding of how memory systems develop during infancy and childhood. ERP studies have documented age-related changes in the patterns of late slow-wave activity that are consistent with the brain-based perspective on memory development in infancy. It remains unclear, however, whether this late slow-wave activity reflects brain activity that is generated in the MTL. Future research will capitalize on advances in source localization techniques to further characterize how changes in the brain drive changes in memory behavior across infancy. Additionally, researchers have begun to use neuroimaging technology with older children to further characterize how changes in the brain are related to the continuing development of explicit memory during childhood.

Conclusions

Neuroscience has long offered developmental psychologists tantalizing glimpses into the potential mechanisms underlying cognitive development. However, it is only recently that the marriage of developmental psychology and cognitive neuroscience has allowed us to test directly models of development in various cognitive domains. The examples provided above illustrate the value added by this approach. By integrating the study of brain and behavioral development, researchers have been able to move beyond simple description of the developmental course of face processing or memory, to a richer understanding of the neurocognitive mechanisms that underlie these developmental changes. Moreover, particularly in the context of face processing, researchers have shown the powerful role of experience in shaping the neural systems that underlie this ability. This in turn raises the possibility that future studies will not focus on brain or behavior, but rather brain and behavior, in which knowledge of the brain informs knowledge of behavior and vice versa.

In our view, other domains of development would equally benefit from this marriage of disciplines. For example, we know a tremendous amount about the development of the prefrontal cortex, which has the potential to inform our understanding of the development of executive functions (for example, see Happaney, Zelazo, & Stuss [2004]). Moving away from cognitive domains, a great deal is now known about the neural systems that underlie different domains of emotional functioning in adults; here we would encourage further elaboration of the nascent field of developmental affective neuroscience. Finally, we should not restrict our knowledge of brain-behavior relations to the study of typically developing children; rather, our understanding of the mechanisms underlying developmental disorders will benefit from a developmental cognitive neuroscience perspective.

Despite making significant contributions to our understanding of cognitive development, the field of developmental cognitive neuroscience is very much in its infancy. Future research should aim to integrate the tools that are available to the developmental cognitive neuroscientist. By combining neurophysiological, neuroimaging and behavioral measures of the same cognitive phenomena, and studying cognitive processes longitudinally, the field will make great gains in resolving the fundamental questions of cognitive development.

Acknowledgment

The writing of this paper was made possible by grants from the NIH (NS32976 and NS32755).

References

Aylward, E.H., Park, J.E., Field, K.M., Parsons, A.C., Richards, T.L., Cramer, S.C., et al. (2005). Brain activation during face perception: Evidence of a developmental change. *Journal of Cognitive Neuroscience, 17,* 308–319.

Bauer, P., Wiebe, S., Carver, L., Waters, J., & Nelson, C. (2003). Developments in long-term explicit memory late in the first year of life: Behavioral and electrophysiological indices. *Psychological Science, 14,* 629–635.

Bentin, S., Allison, T., Puce, A., Perez, E., & McCarthy, G. (1996). Electrophysiological studies of face perception in humans. *Journal of Cognitive Neuroscience, 8,* 551–565.

Carver, L., Bauer, P., & Nelson, C. (2000). Associations between infant brain activity and recall memory. *Developmental Science, 2,* 234–246.

Casey, B., Cohen, J., Jezzard, P., Turner, R., Noll, D., Trainor, R., et al. (1995). Activation of prefrontal cortex in children during a nonspatial working memory task with functional MRI. *Neuroimage, 2,* 221–229.

Cohen, N., Eichenbaum, H., Deacedo, B., & Corkin, S. (1985). Different memory systems underlying acquisition of procedural and declarative knowledge. *Annals of the New York Academy of Sciences, 444,* 54–71.

Cohen, N., & Squire, L. (1980). Preserved learning and retention of pattern analyzing skill in amnesia: Dissociation of knowing how and knowing that. *Science, 10,* 207–209.

Corkin, S. (1968). Acquisition of motor skill after bilateral medial temporal-lobe excision. *Neuropsychologia, 6,* 255–265.

Courchesne, E., Ganz, L., & Norcia, A.M. (1981). Event-related potentials to human faces in infants. *Child Development, 52,* 804–811.

Cycowicz, Y. (2000). Memory development and event-related brain potentials in children. *Biological Psychology, 54,* 145–174.

Cycowicz, Y., Friedman, D., & Duff, M. (2003). Pictures and their colors: What do children remember? *Journal of Cognitive Neuroscience, 15,* 759–768.

Darwin, C. (1872). *The expression of the emotions in man and animals.* London: Murray.

de Haan, M., & Johnson, M.H. (2003). *The cognitive neuroscience of development.* London: Psychology Press.

de Haan, M., Johnson, M.H., & Halit, H. (2003). Development of face-sensitive event-related potentials during infancy: A review. *International Journal of Psychophysiology, 51,* 45–58.

de Haan, M., & Nelson, C. (1997). Recognition of the mother's face by six-month-old infants: A neurobehavioral study. *Child Development, 68,* 187–210.

de Haan, M., & Nelson, C.A. (1999). Brain activity differentiates face and object processing in 6-month-old infants. *Developmental Psychology, 35,* 1113–1121.
de Haan, M., Pascalis, O., & Johnson, M.H. (2002). Specialization of neural mechanisms underlying face recognition in human infants. *Journal of Cognitive Neuroscience, 14,* 199–209.
Desimone, R. (1991). Face-selective cells in the temporal cortex of monkeys. *Journal of Cognitive Neuroscience, 3,* 1–8.
Farah, M.J. (1996). Is face recognition 'special'? Evidence from neuropsychology. *Behavioral Brain Research, 76,* 181–189.
Farah, M.J., Rabinowitz, C., Quinn, G.E., & Liu, G.T. (2000). Early commitment of neural substrates for face recognition. *Cognitive Neuropsychology, 17,* 117–123.
Fischer, K.W. (1987). Relations between brain and cognitive development. *Child Development, 58,* 623–632.
Goldman-Rakic, P.S. (1987). Development of cortical circuitry and cognitive function. *Child Development, 58,* 601–622.
Graf, P., & Schacter, D. (1985). Implicit and explicit memory for new associations in normal and amnesic patients. *Journal of Experimental Psychology: Learning, Memory, and Cognition, 10,* 164–178.
Halit, H., de Haan, M., & Johnson, M.H. (2003). Cortical specialisation for face processing: Face-sensitive event-related potential components in 3- and 12-month-old infants. *Neuroimage, 19,* 1180–1193.
Happaney, K., Zelazo, P.D., & Stuss, D.T. (2004). Development of orbitofrontal function: Current themes and future directions. *Brain and Cognition, 55,* 1–10.
Hartshorn, K., Rovee-Collier, C., Gerhardstein, P., Bhatt, R., Wondoloski, T., Klein, P., et al. (1998). The ontogeny of long-term memory over the first year-and-a-half of life. *Developmental Psychobiology, 32,* 69–89.
Hofmann, M.J., Salapatek, P., & Kuskowski, M. (1981). Evidence for visual memory in the averaged and single evoked potentials of human infants. *Infant Behavior and Development, 4,* 401–421.
Hunt, R., Couperus, J., Nelson, C., & Thomas, K. (2004, June). *Continuous recognition memory in adults and children: An ERP study of parametric memory load manipulation.* Paper presented at the Annual Meeting of the Organization for Human Brain Mapping, Budapest, Hungary.
Itier, R.J., & Taylor, M.J. (2002). Inversion and contrast polarity reversal affect both encoding and recognition processes of unfamiliar faces: A repetition study using ERPs. *Neuroimage, 15,* 353–372.
Johnson, M.H. (1998). The neural basis of cognitive development. In W. Damon (Ed.), *Handbook of child psychology, Vol. 2: Cognition, perception, and language* (pp. 1–49). Hoboken, NJ: Wiley & Sons.
Johnson, M.H., Dziurawiec, S., Ellis, H., & Morton, J. (1991). Newborns' preferential tracking of face-like stimuli and its subsequent decline. *Cognition, 40,* 1–19.
Kanwisher, N. (2000). Domain specificity in face perception. *Nature Neuroscience, 3,* 759–763.
Kanwisher, N., McDermott, J., & Chun, M.M. (1997). The fusiform face area: A module in human extrastriate cortex specialized for face perception. *Journal of Neuroscience, 17,* 4302–4311.
Marshall, D., Drummey, A., Fox, N., & Newcombe, N. (2000). An event-related potential study of item recognition memory in children and adults. *Journal of Cognition and Development, 2,* 210–224.
McCarthy, G., Puce, A., Gore, J.C., & Allison, T. (1997). Face-specific processing in the human fusiform gyrus. *Journal of Cognitive Neuroscience, 9,* 605–610.
McDonough, L., Mandler, J., McKee, R., & Squire, L. (1995). The deferred imitation task as a nonverbal measure of declarative memory. *Proceedings of the National Academy of Science, 92,* 7580–7584.
McKee, R., & Squire, L. (1993). On the development of declarative memory. *Journal of Experimental Psychology: Learning, Memory, and Cognition, 19,* 397–404.
Menon, V., Boyett-Anderson, J., & Reiss, A. (2005). Maturation of medial temporal lobe response and connectivity during memory encoding. *Cognitive Brain Research, 25,* 379–385.
Mondloch, C.J., Geldart, S., Maurer, D., & Le Grand, R. (2003). Developmental changes in face processing skills. *Journal of Experimental Child Psychology, 86,* 67–84.
Mondloch, C.J., Lewis, T.L., Budreau, D.R., Maurer, D., Dannemiller, J.L., Stephens, B.R., et al. (1999). Face perception during early infancy. *Psychological Science, 10,* 419–422.
Nelson, C.A. (1995). The ontogeny of human memory: A cognitive neuroscience perspective. *Developmental Psychology, 31,* 723–738.
Nelson, C.A. (1997). Electrophysiological correlates of memory development in the first year of life. In H. Reese & M. Franzen (Eds.), *Biological and neuropsychological mechanisms: Life-span developmental psychology* (pp. 95–132). Mahwah, NJ: Erlbaum Associates.
Nelson, C.A. (2001). The development and neural bases of face recognition. *Infant and Child Development, 10,* 3–18.
Nelson, C.A., & Bloom, F.E. (1997). Child development and neuroscience. *Child Development, 68,* 970–987.

Nelson, C.A., & Collins, K. (1991). Event-related potential and looking time analysis of infants' responses to familiar and novel events: Implications for visual recognition memory. *Developmental Psychology, 27,* 50–58.
Nelson, C.A., & Collins, P. (1992). Neural and behavioral correlates of visual recognition in 4- and 8-month-old infants. *Brain and Cognition, 19,* 105–121.
Nelson, C.A., de Haan, M., & Thomas, K.M. (2006). Neural bases of cognitive development. In W. Damon, R. Lerner, D. Kuhn & R. Siegler (Eds.), *Handbook of child psychology (6th ed.), Vol. 2: Cognition, perception and language.* Hoboken. N.J.: Wiley & Sons.
Nelson, C.A., Luciana, M. (Eds.) (2001). *Handbook of developmental cognitive neuroscience.* Cambridge, MA: MIT Press.
Nelson, C.A., & Salapatek, P. (1986). Electrophysiological correlates of infant recognition memory. *Child Development, 57,* 1483–1497.
Passarotti, A.M., Paul, B.M., Bussiere, J.R., Buxton, R.B., Wong, E.C., & Stiles, J. (2003). The development of face and location processing: An fMRI study. *Developmental Science, 6,* 100–117.
Reynolds, G., & Richards, J. (2005). Familiarization, attention, and recognition memory in infancy: An event-related potential and cortical source localization study. *Developmental Psychology, 41,* 598–615.
Richards, J. (2003). Attention affects the recognition of briefly presented visual stimuli in infants: An ERP study. *Developmental Science, 6,* 312–328.
Rossion, B., Delvenne, J.F., Debatisse, D., Goffaux, V., Bruyer, R., Crommelinck, M., et al. (1999). Spatio-temporal localization of the face inversion effect: An event-related potentials study. *Biological Psychology, 50,* 173–189.
Rossion, B., Gauthier, I., Tarr, M.J., Despland, P., Bruyer, R., Linotte, S., et al. (2000). The N170 occipito-temporal component is delayed and enhanced to inverted faces but not to inverted objects: An electrophysiological account of face-specific processes in the human brain. *Neuroreport, 11,* 69–74.
Rovee-Collier, C. (1997). Dissociations in infant memory: Rethinking the development of implicit and explicit memory. *Psychological Review, 104,* 467–498.
Rovee-Collier, C., Hayne, H., & Colombo, M. (2001). *The development of implicit and explicit memory.* Amsterdam: Benjamins.
Schacter, D., & Moscovitch, M. (1984). Infants, amnesics, and dissociable memory systems. In M. Moscovitch (Ed.), *Advances in the study of communication and affect* (Vol. 9, pp. 173–216). New York: Plenum Press.
Scott, L., & Nelson, C.A. (2004). The developmental neurobiology of face processing. In B.J. Casey (Ed.), *Review of psychiatry series* (Vol. 23, pp. 29–68). Washington, DC: American Psychiatric Publishing.
Scoville, W. (1968). Amnesia after bilateral mesial temporal-lobe excision: Introduction to case H.M. *Neuropsychologia, 6,* 211–213.
Scoville, W., & Milner, B. (1957). Loss of recent memory after bilateral hippocampal lesions. *Journal of Neurology, Neurosurgery, and Psychiatry, 20,* 11–21.
Seress, L. (2001). Morphological changes of the human hippocampal formation from midgestation to early childhood. In C. Nelson & M. Luciana (Eds.), *Handbook of developmental cognitive neuroscience.* Cambridge, MA: MIT Press.
Seress, L., & Ribak, C. (1995). Postnatal development of CA3 pyramidal neurons and their afferents in the Ammon's horn of rhesus monkeys. *Hippocampus, 5,* 217–231.
Squire, L. (1994). Declarative and nondeclarative memory: Multiple brain systems supporting learning and memory. In D. Schacter & E. Tulving (Eds.), *Memory systems 1994* (pp. 203–231). Cambridge, MA: MIT Press.
Tarr, M.J., & Gauthier, I. (2000). FFA: A flexible fusiform area for subordinate-level visual processing automatized by expertise. *Nature Neuroscience, 3,* 764–769.
Taylor, M.J., Batty, M., & Itier, R.J. (2004). The faces of development: A review of early face processing over childhood. *Journal of Cognitive Neuroscience, 16,* 1426–1442.
Thomas, K., Hunt, R., Townsend, E., Couperus, J., Nelson, C., & Mueller, B. (2004, June). *Developmental differences in continuous recognition memory: An fMRI study of medial temporal lobe function.* Paper presented at the Annual Meeting of the Organization for Human Brain Mapping, Budapest, Hungary.
Tzourio-Mazoyer, N., De Schonen, S., Crivello, F., Reutter, B., Aujard, Y., & Mazoyer, B. (2002). Neural correlates of woman face processing by 2-month-old infants. *Neuroimage, 15,* 454–461.
Webb, S.J., Long, J.D., & Nelson, C.A. (2005). A longitudinal investigation of visual event-related potentials in the first year of life. *Developmental Science, 8,* 605–616.

Paper

Human Development 2006;49:273–293
DOI: 10.1159/000095580

Human Development

Identifying the Neural Correlates Underlying Social Pain: Implications for Developmental Processes

Naomi I. Eisenberger

University of California, Los Angeles, Calif., USA

Key Words
Anterior cingulate cortex · Attachment · Neuroimaging · Pain processes · Social pain

Abstract
Although the need for social connection is critical for early social development as well as for psychological well-being throughout the lifespan, relatively little is known about the neural processes involved in maintaining social connections. The following review summarizes what is known regarding the neural correlates underlying feeling of 'social pain', the painful experiences associated with social estrangement or loss, which may be critical for motivating social connection. Using this general framework, the review then specifies the ways in which neuroimaging may provide insight into the development of these neural systems in humans. To this end, the review elaborates on the specific types of questions that are best addressed using neuroimaging techniques and examines several lines of inquiry within the developmental literature that may be aided by these methods.
Copyright © 2006 S. Karger AG, Basel

We need others. We need others to love and we need to be loved by them. There is no doubt that without it, we too, like the infant left alone, would cease to grow, cease to develop...
Leo Buscaglia

Few would question the assertion that children need care and affection for successful growth and development. Although this statement seems self-evident today, psychologists long thought otherwise. Until 50 years ago, it was believed that a child's bond to his or her caregiver was based solely on the child's need for food and the

KARGER

Fax +41 61 306 12 34
E-Mail karger@karger.ch
www.karger.com

© 2006 S. Karger AG, Basel
0018–716X/06/0495–0273$23.50/0

Accessible online at:
www.karger.com/hde

Naomi I. Eisenberger, Department of Psychiatry and Biobehavioral Sciences, University of California
Los Angeles, CA 90095-7076 (USA)
Tel. +1 310 825 2576, Fax +1 310 794 9247
E-Mail neisenbe@ucla.edu

caregiver's ability to fulfill that basic need [Dollard & Miller, 1950; Mussen & Conger, 1956]. In one of the most profound demonstrations to the contrary, Harlow [1958] and Harlow and Zimmermann [1959] showed that infant rhesus monkeys preferred a cloth surrogate mother that provided them with contact comfort to a wire mesh mother that provided them with food, indicating the existence of a need for social connection, over and above the need for food.

As further evidence of the profound importance of social connection, individuals who lack social connection early in life are likely to show disrupted social and emotional development. For example, in Harlow's classic studies, infant rhesus monkeys, raised without the companionship of a real or a cloth mother, exhibited significant behavioral and emotional problems [Harlow, 1958; Harlow & Zimmerman, 1959]. Although the initial reason for raising infant monkeys in isolation was to investigate the development of specific learning skills without the distraction of mother-infant interactions, the extreme emotional disturbances seen among these isolated infants soon led Harlow and others to focus their investigations on the emotional consequences of early maternal separation instead [Harlow, Harlow, & Suomi, 1971; Pollak, 2005].

Paralleling Harlow's work in primates, Bowlby's [1969] influential theory of attachment, which outlined the adaptive significance of the mother-infant relationship, was built upon observations that children who were separated from their primary caregivers early in life exhibited severe distress during the separation episode as well as continued psychological disturbance following reunion. From these observations, Bowlby suggested that prolonged separation from a caregiver in early life was likely to lead to various forms of psychopathology in later life. Indeed, recent observations from Eastern European orphanages support this claim; orphans lacking early social ties do not develop normal social or emotional skills and have long-lasting problems maintaining social relationships [Wismer Fries & Pollak, 2004].

Despite the well-known importance of early social ties for normal growth and development, relatively little is known about the underlying neural systems that regulate these attachment-related processes in humans or how these systems may be altered by early negative experiences. Given the profound influence that social ties have on psychological function, both in childhood and throughout the lifespan [Repetti, Taylor, & Seeman, 2002], it is important to investigate how the systems involved in maintaining social connection develop, how they may influence or interact with the activity and function of other systems and how they may become altered through negative experiences.

The following review will begin by summarizing what is known regarding the neural correlates underlying feelings of social estrangement in adult humans (for a comprehensive review of the neural correlates underlying feelings of social connection and affiliative motivation, see Depue & Morrone-Strupinsky [2005]). Although little is known about the neural underpinnings of human social attachment processes per se (however, see Gillath, Bunge, Shaver, Wendelken, & Mikulincer [2005], Schore [2000]), recent research has begun to elucidate some of the neurocognitive correlates underlying feelings of 'social pain' [Eisenberger & Lieberman, 2004], the hurt feelings following social rejection [Eisenberger, Lieberman, & Williams, 2003] or social loss [Gundel, O'Connor, Littrell, Fort, & Lane, 2003; Najib, Lorberbaum, Kose, Bohning, & George, 2004]. Experiences of social pain may be critical in maintaining attachment relationships, as the pain of social distance may motivate distress-related behaviors in infants and young children (e.g., crying) as well as maternal behaviors (e.g., retrieval of infants), both of which are aimed at preventing social estrangement. Moreover, the neural circuitry supporting socially painful experience may be critically important during early development when individuals cannot fully take care of themselves and are almost exclusively dependent upon others for survival. This review will outline some of the work that has investigated the neurocognitive correlates of social pain in humans as well as related work that has investigated attachment-related behaviors in animals.

Using this general framework for understanding some of the neural structures involved in avoiding social distance and maintaining social connection, this review will then specify the ways in which neuroimaging may provide insight into the development of these neural systems in humans. In the past decade, functional magnetic resonance imaging has been increasingly used as a noninvasive technique for investigating the neural underpinnings of specific social processes, such as those that underlie emotion regulation, person perception and empathy [Adolphs, 2003; Blakemore, Winston, & Frith, 2004; Lieberman, in press; Ochsner, 2004]. However, despite the fact that one of the primary goals of most of these psychological processes is to establish, navigate and maintain social relationships, relatively little work has focused on the neural correlates associated with feelings of social connection or social estrangement. Moreover, at this point, no work in humans has investigated the *development* of the neural structures that underlie feelings of social connection or estrangement or how early social experiences may alter the functioning of this neural circuitry. Given the importance of social relationships for social development and long-term psychological health, developmental psychologists and developmental neuroscientists are poised to play a critical role in helping to understand the developing social brain. To this end, this review will elaborate on the specific types of questions that are best addressed using neuroimaging and will examine several lines of inquiry within the developmental literature that may be significantly illuminated by these methods.

Social Pain and Its Neural Underpinnings

> 'A condition that makes being a mammal so painful is separation from a sustaining member or members of a group' [MacLean, 1985b, p. 220].

As noted by MacLean, one of the consequences of being human, or of being a mammal more generally, is the profound experience of pain when separated from loved ones. Indeed, the English language is replete with phrases that denote the pain associated with broken social bonds. We complain of '*hurt* feelings' and '*broken* hearts' to describe feelings of social pain and, notably, we have few ways to express these feelings other than with words denoting physical pain [MacDonald & Leary, 2005]. Why is it that broken social ties have the capacity to 'wound' us so deeply?

One mechanism that could explain why social separation is experienced as painful follows from the importance of close social ties for survival in mammalian species [Eisenberger & Lieberman, 2004; MacDonald & Leary, 2005]. Mammals are unique in their need for prolonged attention from a caregiver. Unlike our reptilian ancestors, who are born almost completely mature and self-sufficient [MacLean, 1985a], mammals require close contact with a caregiver in order to acquire the appropriate nourishment and protection to survive. Because of this, separation of the infant from the caregiver is a dangerous proposition that may result in death for the infant. Consequently, it has been hypothesized that the social attachment system, the system that keeps us near close others, may have piggybacked onto the physical pain system to promote survival in mammalian species [Panksepp, 1998]. Thus, to the extent that being separated from a caregiver is dangerous, feeling pain in response to this separation may be an adaptive way to prevent it.

This hypothesized overlap in the systems underlying physical and social pain was first proposed by Panksepp [1998] based on some work examining the effect of exogenous opiates on pain tolerance in puppies. Panksepp noted that, in addition to reducing pain experience, opiate administration also reduced crying behavior in puppies that were socially isolated [Panksepp, Herman, Conner, Bishop, & Scott, 1978]. Others have found similar effects, showing that morphine, an opiate-based drug, reduced separation-induced distress vocalizations in nonhuman primates as well [Kalin, Shelton, & Barksdale, 1988]. From this, it has been suggested that opioid mechanisms may be one neural substrate common to both physical and social pain [Nelson & Panksepp, 1998; reviewed in Panksepp, 1998].

Recent evidence from neuroimaging studies provides further support for this hypothesized overlap by showing that some of the same neural structures involved in the experience of physical pain are also involved in the distressing experience associated with social rejection or social loss. Moreover, animal studies have shown that this same neural circuitry also plays a role in specific behaviors that are critical for maintaining mother-infant contact such as maternal care as well as distress vocalizations, emitted by infants when separated from the mother to reestablish social contact. Thus, there may be certain neural structures that are involved both in feelings of social distress upon social separation and in initiating behaviors aimed at reestablishing contact with close others.

I will first review some evidence linking activity in the dorsal portion of the anterior cingulate cortex (dACC) to feelings of physical and social pain in humans. (In the second half of the paper, I will review another account of the function of this neural region, namely its role in conflict monitoring [Botvinick, Cohen, & Carter, 2004].) I will also review other studies in adult humans that have explored the neural correlates underlying feelings of social pain. These studies will reveal the involvement of other neural structures in the experience and regulation of social pain, including the insula, involved in the processing of visceral sensation as well as negative affective experience [Aziz, Schnitzler, & Enck, 2000; Cechetto & Saper, 1987; Lane, Reiman, Ahern, Schwartz, & Davidson, 1997; Phan, Wager, Taylor, & Liberzon, 2004; Philips et al., 1997], the periaqueductal gray (PAG), involved in pain processing and attachment-related behaviors [Bandler & Shipley, 1994; Dunckley et al., 2005], and the right ventral prefrontal cortex (RVPFC), involved in regulating the distress of physical pain or negative affect more generally [Hariri, Bookheimer, & Mazziota, 2000; Lieberman, Hariri, Jarcho, Eisenberger, & Bookheimer, 2005; Petrovic & Ingvar, 2002]. Lastly, I will review some of the animal literature linking the anterior cingulate gyrus and the PAG to attachment-related behaviors more generally.

Defining Social Pain

Throughout this review, the term 'social pain' will be used broadly to refer to the distressing experience that results from perceived social separation. In the same manner that 'separation distress' can be defined as the distressing experience resulting from perceived distance from a caregiver [Bowlby, 1969], social pain can be defined as *the distressing experience arising from the perception of psychological distance from close others or from the social group.* In this case, psychological distance can include perceptions of rejection, exclusion, noninclusion, loss or any socially relevant cue that makes an individual feel disconnected from or disregarded by relationship partners. Whereas infants may only be capable of detecting actual physical distance from a caregiver, emergent cognitive capacities soon enable young children to monitor not only objective distance from the caregiver, but also perceived psychological distance from the caregiver, an assessment that relies on a more complex understanding of sociorelational information.

Based on expanding cognitive capacities that allow adults to represent, manipulate, imagine and predict complex social information, many more cues may be capable of eliciting social pain in adults than are capable of eliciting separation distress in infants. For example, human adults can experience social pain not only based on the perception of psychological distance from an individual, but also based on the perception of psychological distance from a *social group*, a more complex mental representation. In addition, human adults can experience social pain or anxiety at the mere *possibility* of social distance. The capacity to represent complex ideas such as 'the social group' or 'the possibility of social distance' may only be possible in later stages of development with the emergence of enhanced cognitive resources that allow symbolic and propositional representations [Brothers, 1990; Deacon, 1997; Lieberman, Gaunt, Gilbert, & Trope, 2002].

It should also be noted that the social pain resulting from perceived distance from a caregiver, attachment figure or significant other (e.g., separation distress) may be phenomenologically and neurocognitively different from the social pain resulting from perceived distance from one's social group or peers (e.g., social rejection). For example, it has been shown that the neural systems underlying separation-induced distress vocalizations are dissociable from the neural systems underlying threat-induced (e.g., perception of novel stimuli) freezing behavior in primates [A.S. Fox et al., 2005; Kalin & Shelton, 1998]. Thus, it is possible that being rejected by one's peers may be processed as a threatening environmental stressor rather than as a separation-related stressor and should therefore recruit neural systems related to threat perception rather than separation perception. However, based on similar neural activations to social rejection from peers and to the loss of significant others in adult humans [Eisenberger et al., 2003; Gundel et al., 2003; Najib et al., 2004], the term 'social pain' will be used to refer to both types of experiences for the purposes of the present review. Further research will be needed to better understand the extent to which experiences of social rejection and experiences of social loss rely on similar or distinct neural systems and whether there are developmental changes in the neural systems that underlie these experiences.

Physical and Social Pain in Humans

In humans, the dACC plays a role both in the unpleasantness of physical pain as well as in the distress associated with social estrangement. With regard to physical pain, the dACC seems to be involved in the *affective* as opposed to the *sensory* component of pain. For example, following cingulotomy for chronic pain, a procedure in which a portion of the anterior cingulate cortex is removed, patients report still being able to feel the intensity of pain but report that the pain no longer bothers them [Foltz & White, 1968], highlighting the role that this structure plays in registering the distressing, rather than the purely sensory, component of the pain experience. In line with this, several neuroimaging studies have shown that the activity of the dACC corresponds to perceived pain unpleasantness, whereas the activity of the primary somatosensory cortex corresponds to perceived pain intensity from cutaneous stimulation [Peyron, Laurent, & Garcia-Larrea, 2000; Ploghaus et al., 1999; Rainville, Duncan, Price, Carrier, & Bushnell, 1997; Sawamoto et al., 2000]. The insula, another neural region involved in pain experience, processes visceral rather than cutaneous sensation; its specific role in the affective versus sensory dimension of pain is not yet clear [Aziz et al., 2000].

More recent research has begun to reveal the role of the dACC in the distress of social pain as well. In a study investigating the neural correlates of social exclusion [Eisenberger et al., 2003], participants were led to believe that they would be playing a virtual ball-tossing game called Cyberball [Williams, Cheung, & Choi, 2000], with two other players over the internet while in the functional magnetic resonance imaging scanner. Upon being excluded from the game, compared to when being included, participants showed increased activity in a region of the dACC, very similar to the region of the dACC associated with the unpleasantness of physical pain. Moreover, the magnitude of dACC activity correlated strongly ($r = 0.88$) with self-reports of social distress felt during the exclusion episode (e.g., 'I felt rejected,' 'I felt invisible'), such that individuals who showed greater dACC activity in response to social rejection also reported feeling more distressed by the rejection episode. Participants also showed increased activity in the insula, a region known to be involved in processing visceral sensation (e.g., visceral pain) as well as negative affective states [Aziz et al., 2000; Cechetto & Saper, 1987; Lane et al., 1997; Phan et al., 2004; Philips et al., 1997]; however, insular activity did not correlate significantly with self-reported social distress in this study.

Lastly, participants also showed increased activity in the RVPFC, a region of the brain typically associated with regulating feelings of pain or negative affect [Hariri et al., 2000; Lieberman et al., 2005; Petrovic & Ingvar, 2002]. Moreover, greater activity in the RVPFC was associated with lower levels of self-reported social distress in response to the ball-tossing game ($r = -0.69$), suggesting that this region may have been playing a role in regulating the distress of being socially excluded.

A similar study investigated how neural responses to social rejection (using the same exclusion paradigm described in the previous study) related to real-world feelings of social connection or estrangement in daily social interactions. It was found that individuals who showed greater activity in the dACC, PAG and amygdala in response to a single episode of social rejection in the scanner were more likely to report feeling socially disconnected during their daily social interactions across a 10-day period [Eisenberger, Gable, & Lieberman, 2006]. Thus, in addition to the dACC, activity in the PAG and amygdala may also relate to socially painful experience in humans.

Although the role of the PAG in social pain processing fits with previous work relating this neural region to pain processing as well as attachment-related behaviors in nonhuman mammals (distress vocalizations; nursing behavior [Bandler & Shipley, 1994; Dunckley et al., 2005; Lonstein & Stern, 1998]), the role of the amygdala in social pain processes has not yet been clearly established. Animal research has demonstrated that amygdala lesions consistently reduce fearfulness to innate fear stimuli (e.g., replicas of snakes), but have no clear effects on social fears [Amaral, 2003]. Amygdala lesions can either produce no changes in social behavior, decreases in social fear or increases in social fear, depending on the age at which the lesion occurred (i.e., lesions during infancy lead to increased social fear, lesions during adulthood lead to reduced social fear [Amaral, 2003]). In addition, increased amygdala activity in nonhuman primates correlates negatively with separation-induced distress vocalizations, thought to be indicative of social pain processes [A.S. Fox et al., 2005; Kalin & Shelton, 1998], suggesting that amygdala activation may be associated with reduced social pain experience. Thus, it is possible that the amygdala is more involved in signaling when a social situation might be threatening or socially painful than in the actual experience of social pain per se. Future work is needed to determine the extent to which the amygdala plays a role in social pain processes.

Other studies have investigated the neural correlates associated with more personally relevant forms of social pain. In one study, bereaved participants were scanned while viewing pictures of their deceased first-degree relative or a stranger. In response to viewing pictures of the deceased, compared to pictures of a stranger, the participants showed greater activity in regions of the dACC and insula [Gundel et al., 2003]. Similarly, in a study investigating the neural responses associated with grieving a romantic relationship, women whose romantic relationship had ended within the preceding 4 months showed greater activity in several neural regions when thinking about their relationship, compared to when thinking about another individual, including the dACC [Najib et al., 2004]. However, there were many neural regions activated in response to thinking about the former partner, and thus it is difficult to clearly identify which neural activations are specifically related to feelings of social pain.

Lastly, several studies have examined the neural structures involved in human parental behavior. Two of these studies scanned mothers while they listened to baby cries versus control sounds (white noise), a contrast which might lead to greater feelings of social distress and more attachment-related behaviors (e.g., attempts at soothing the infant). Results indicated that mothers had more dACC activity to infant cries compared to white noise [Lorberbaum et al., 1999, 2002], consistent with the animal data demonstrating the cingulate's involvement in the caregiver's response to distress vocalizations [MacLean, 1985a, 1985b; MacLean & Newman, 1988; Stamm, 1955]. Mothers also showed greater activity across several different prefrontal cortical regions in response to hearing baby cries as well, including the medial prefrontal cortex, RVPFC and dorsolateral prefrontal cortex. Given previous work showing the involvement of the RVPFC as well as the medial prefrontal cortex [Quirk, Likhtik, Pelletier, & Pare, 2003] in regulating limbic activity or negative affective processes, it is possible that these activations were associated with mothers' attempts to regulate their own distress at hearing infant cries; however, this account is only speculative. Additional studies are needed to more carefully determine the types of emotional experiences that are associated with these neural activations.

An additional study scanned mothers and fathers of young children as well as men and women without children while they listened to infant crying and laughing [Seifritz et al., 2003]. When comparing neural activity while listening to infant cries versus infant laughing, parents (mothers and fathers) showed greater activity in the right amygdala, middle cingulate cortex, bilateral insulae and the left ventral prefrontal cortex than nonparents. This study extends previous findings by showing that similar patterns of neural activity are found for mothers as well as fathers while hearing infant cries.

Based on a prior, influential review suggesting that the dACC is involved in cognitive processing, whereas the rostral-ventral division of the ACC is involved in affective processing [Bush, Luu, & Posner, 2000], it may be surprising that many of the studies that have examined social pain processes in adult humans have found activity in the dorsal, rather than the rostral, ACC. It should be noted that at the time that this prior review was conducted, no studies of social pain processes had been conducted. Moreover, this review did not include or integrate any of the studies showing that physical pain, which seems more affective than cognitive in nature, primarily activates regions of the dACC [Peyron et al, 2000]. Thus, this proposed distinction between dACC and rostral division of the ACC may need some updating and reformulation based on the addition of the physical pain studies as well as the new studies of affective processes that have been conducted since that time (for a possible alternative account, see Eisenberger & Lieberman [2004]).

Attachment-Related Behaviors in Nonhuman Mammals

Animal work has focused less on the painful experiences associated with social separation and more on the behaviors involved in preventing social separation and promoting social contact. Mammals, unique in their profound need for social contact, engage in certain behaviors aimed at maintaining social bonds, including maternal care (e.g., nursing, pup retrieval) and audiovocal communication for maintaining mother-offspring contact [MacLean, 1985a, 1993]. Both of these behaviors aid in maintaining mother-infant contact, either by mother-initiated behaviors, such as pup retrieval, or by infant-initiated behaviors, such as the production of distress vocalizations, emitted by separated infants to motivate retrieval by the mother.

The cingulate gyrus, which has no clear counterpart in the reptilian brain, appears for the first time, phylogenetically, in mammalian species [MacLean, 1985a, 1993] and thus may play a role in these uniquely mammalian social behaviors. Research from the animal literature supports this claim. Ablation of the cingulate gyrus in adult female rats results in deficits in maternal behavior, including the nursing and retrieval of pups [Stamm, 1955]. Following cingulate ablation in females, rat mothers become less responsive to the distress vocalizations of their pups. The survival rate of rat pups, whose mothers have cingulate lesions, is only 12%, compared to 95% among healthy controls. This rather dismal survival rate highlights the importance of this structure in maintaining mother-infant contact and promoting the survival of mammalian infants.

In addition to maternal care, the cingulate gyrus also plays a role in the production of distress vocalizations, which are considered to be the most primitive and basic mammalian vocalizations with the original purpose of maintaining mother-infant contact [Lorberbaum et al., 1999, 2002; MacLean, 1985a]. Thus, ablation of the ACC in squirrel monkeys leads to decreased distress vocalizations [Kirzinger & Jurgens, 1982; MacLean & Newman, 1988], whereas electrical stimulation of the ACC leads to the spontaneous production of distress vocalizations in rhesus monkeys [Jurgens & Ploog, 1970; Ploog, 1981; Smith, 1945].

In addition to playing a role in behaviors aimed at maintaining social connection, the dACC also seems to be affected by early social experiences and thus may play a role in the developmental consequences of early negative social experience. For example, maternal separation among newborn rodents changes various neurotransmitter fiber systems in the dACC of these rodents, which can then have consequences for the function of these neural systems [Braun, Lange, Metzger, & Poeggel, 2000]. Conversely, hearing the sound of the mother's voice while being separated buffers against these changes [Braun & Poeggel, 2001; Ziabreva, Schnabel, Poeggel, & Braun, 2003]. Thus, social separation may have the capacity to alter the structural makeup of the neural systems involved in maintaining social bonds, thus enhancing the risk for later socioemotional problems.

Another neural region that has been shown to play a role in attachment-related behaviors in nonhuman mammals is the PAG. The PAG is a small brainstem structure involved in pain processing, maternal behavior and distress vocalizations in nonhuman mammals [Bandler & Shipley, 1994; Dunckley et al., 2005]. In addition, the PAG receives dense projections from the dACC and insular cortex, both of which are activated in response to physical and social pain in humans. Animal studies have shown that lesions to specific regions of the PAG disrupt the nursing posture of rat mothers, resulting in 10% less weight gain in pups of lesioned compared to nonlesioned mothers [Lonstein & Stern, 1998]. Moreover, lesioning the PAG decreases distress vocalizations in pups separated from their mothers, whereas electrically stimulating this region can lead to the spontaneous production of these vocalizations [Panksepp, 1998].

Together, these findings from the human and animal literature suggest that the ACC and PAG are involved in the experience of separation distress as well as in some of the behaviors needed to maintain close social contact with a caregiver or the social group.

In humans, activity in the dACC in response to social estrangement can be thought to index the magnitude of distress felt in response to social estrangement. Activity of the PAG may be indexing a similar type of experience. Moreover, activity in the RVPFC, involved in regulating feelings of social distress or negative affect more generally, can be thought to index regulatory processes. Activity in the insula seems to occur, in some cases, to socially painful experience; however, its role in social pain experience is not yet clear as it has not yet been shown to correlate with the distress of social estrangement. The role of the amygdala in social pain processes is not yet clear either, showing, in some cases, a negative correlation with separation distress (distress vocalizations [A.S. Fox et al., 2005; Kalin & Shelton, 1998]) and in other cases a positive correlation with social pain experience (feelings of social distress during real-world social interactions [Eisenberger et al., 2006]). Although there are undoubtedly many other neural structures involved in maintaining social connections, this review will focus primarily on how activity in these particular neural structures may underlie or contribute to specific developmental issues. In the next section, I will specify the general types of questions that are best addressed using neuroimaging techniques. To illustrate these questions, I will use examples that are based on the neural structures reviewed above and will explore several developmental questions, which may be better understood through the use of neuroimaging techniques.

What Is Neuroimaging Good for?

In the past decade, the field of psychology has witnessed a surge in the number of studies using neuroimaging techniques to elucidate the neural underpinnings of various psychological phenomena. These efforts, however, have been met with varied responses. Some have applauded these techniques, deeming them necessary for generating new ways of understanding psychological experience and treating psychological disorders. These proponents have suggested that neuroimaging techniques afford researchers a better sense of the computational subcomponents that comprise certain psychological experiences and thus may be helpful in determining the specific processes that are altered as a function of psychological disorders. Others have remained more skeptical, arguing that these methods are no better than the ones that researchers have been using for years. These skeptics have suggested that neuroimaging techniques do not provide any additional information that cannot be gleaned from carefully planned behavioral studies and that the scanner itself constrains what can actually be examined with these techniques, as subjects in these studies are limited in what they can physically do within the scanner (e.g., subjects cannot talk or move). In truth, both of these perspectives are valid.

Neuroimaging techniques, like any of the other tools employed for investigating psychological phenomena, are useful for investigating some aspects of psychological experience and not as useful for investigating others [Kosslyn, 1999]. However, within the time span that neuroimaging techniques have been utilized, most researchers have agreed on at least a few very powerful uses for this machinery. These recognized uses for neuroimaging techniques include: (1) determining to what extent seemingly different psychological processes recruit *common* neurocognitive substrates, (2) determining to what extent seemingly similar psychological processes recruit *distinct* neurocognitive substrates and (3) identifying the specific neurocognitive mechanisms underlying complex behavioral and emotional outcomes. In addition, using neuroimaging techniques for examining psychological phenomena moves researchers one step closer to a common language (e.g., neural activity) for understanding psychological experience across disparate levels of analysis (e.g., human, primate, rodent). This use of a common language may promote translational advances that bridge across various disciplines of psychology.

In the next section, I will examine each of these uses for neuroimaging in turn and will elaborate on some developmental questions that may be addressed using these techniques. I will also expand on the ways in which research on social development can be shaped based on recent findings from the neuroimaging literature.

Different Psychological Processes, Similar Neural Substrates

One of the most significant uses for neuroimaging techniques is in determining whether certain psychological phenomena rely on similar neural substrates. Showing that two seemingly different psychological processes activate similar neural regions suggests that these two processes share at least some similar computational mechanisms. Moreover, demonstrating that certain psychological processes share computational similarities may highlight new ways of understanding these processes and may provide new testable hypotheses regarding this shared circuitry.

Physical Pain and Social Pain. Showing that social pain activates some of the same neural regions that are activated by physical pain suggests real, rather than merely metaphorical, similarities between these two processes. For example, in a recent behavioral study examining some potential consequences of this physical-social pain overlap, we investigated whether individuals who are more sensitive to physical pain are also more sensitive to social pain, based on a lower threshold for activity in this same neural system [Eisenberger, Jarcho, Lieberman, & Naliboff, in press]. We found that individuals who at baseline were more sensitive to physical pain (e.g., heat stimulation applied to the forearm) also reported feeling more social distress in response to being socially rejected during a Cyberball game. Moreover, this relationship remained significant after controlling for neuroticism, suggesting that this relationship cannot be easily explained by a general tendency to experience anxiety and thus report higher levels of both types of pain.

Findings such as these may have important implications for understanding the relationships between negative social experiences and physical pain experience. For example, a recent meta-analysis revealed that adults with chronic pain conditions are more likely to have been abused or neglected as children [Davis, Luecken, & Zautra, 2005], pointing to the possibility of a pain-distress system that has become sensitized in part, due to early negative social experience. Moreover, adults with chronic pain disorders, compared to healthy controls, are more likely to have an anxious attachment style, characterized by a heightened sense of concern with a partner's relationship commitment [Ciechanowski, Sullivan, Jensen, Romano, & Summers, 2003], again highlighting the relationship between heightened physical pain experience and a heightened sensitivity to some forms of social pain. Based on these findings, it is possible that treatments for pain disorders may be improved by focusing, not only on the pain symptoms themselves, but also on the social stressors that may exacerbate painful experience.

With regard to developmental issues, the relationship between physical and social pain may have implications for understanding some recent work showing that children who are victimized by their peers report greater levels of physical symptoms, such as headaches and upset stomaches [Nishina, Juvonen, & Witkow, 2005; Williams, Chambers, Logan, & Robinson, 1996]. Although it is possible that peer victimization may increase the risk for physical illness through traditional stress-related physiological processes, such as increases in stress-related hormones that make physical illness more likely [McEwen, 2000], it is also possible that social pain experience can heighten sensitivity to physical pain directly by sensitizing the underlying neural system that supports both types of pain experience. Thus, to the extent that physical and social pain experiences rely on some of the same neural structures for their operation, experiences of social pain may have direct implications for physical pain experience.

Conflict Monitoring and Social Pain. Many studies have suggested that the dACC is involved in 'conflict monitoring', the process of detecting conflicts or discrepancies in incoming information (for a broader review of this account as well as other accounts of dACC function, see Botvinick et al. [2004]). Although conflict monitoring was originally conceptualized as pertaining primarily to behavioral response conflict (when two behavioral tendencies are simultaneously activated), it has now been expanded to include other forms of conflict as well, such as discrepancies between automatic responses and current goals, between actual and expected events, or between new stimuli and preexisting representations that do not map onto each other [Barch et al., 2001; Botvinick, Braver, Barch, Carter, & Cohen, 2001; Botvinick et al., 2004; Braver, Barch, Gray, Molfese, & Snyder, 2001; Hajcak, Holroyd, Moser, & Simons, 2005; Inui et al., 2000; MacLeod & MacDonald, 2000]. Once a conflict has been detected, regions of the lateral prefrontal cortex, including, in some cases, the RVPFC, are recruited in order to exert top-down controlled processes to resolve the conflict [Carter et al., 2000; MacDonald, Cohen, Stenger, & Carter, 2000].

Notably, our own research has shown that dACC activity in response to errors, one form of conflict (when behavioral responses conflict with current goals), during a simple cognitive task (go/no-go), overlapped with dACC activity in response to social rejection [Eisenberger & Lieberman, 2006], suggesting that conflict detection and social pain processes may rely on some of the same computational substrates. Based on this possible functional overlap in the neural substrates underlying conflict detection and social pain processes, as well as the suggestion that this neurocognitive loop is critical for the development of affect and behavioral regulation in children [Casey et al., 1997], it is important to understand how these processes, which seem quite distinct, relate to one another.

Research has suggested that conflict monitoring processes become more efficient with increasing age [Casey et al., 1997]. Based on the overlap in the neural structures underlying conflict detection processes and social distress responses, several questions can be asked. For example, if it is the case that conflict detection processes show increasing efficiency during adolescence [Davies, Segalowitz, & Gavin, 2004; Ladouceur, Dahl, & Carter, 2004], it is interesting to note that this increasing efficiency seems to parallel the heightened sensitivity to peer evaluation that accompanies this time period. Does the development of more efficient conflict detection processes make individuals more sensitive to rejection? Are individuals who are less concerned with social connection also less sensitive to conflict more generally? Furthermore, does the ability to regulate negative emotional responses to social rejection relate to the capacity to resolve conflict? What would such findings imply for the development of affect and behavioral regulatory processes?

While these findings open up many more questions than answers, they also provide some novel ways of thinking about the complex relationships between the development of cognitive and social skills and the ways in which these processes may influence one another. In response to some of the questions listed above, preliminary evidence suggests that individuals who are unconcerned with social relationships show reduced neural activity in response to errors [Santesso, Segalowitz, & Schmidt, 2005], suggesting that reduced social sensitivity may relate to less efficient conflict or error detection processes. Another study has shown that experimentally manipulating social pressures can alter neural responses to errors, specifically the error-related negativity [Hajcak, Moser, Yeung, & Simons, 2005], an event-related brain potential observed when errors are committed, which has been localized to the ACC [Holroyd, Dien, & Coles, 1998]. In this study, participants performed a conflict detection task while either being evaluated (e.g., told that a research assistant was viewing their responses and comparing them to how others did at the same task) or while not being evaluated. Results showed that subjects showed larger error-related negativities to errors when they were being evaluated than when they were not, suggesting that social stressors may influence sensitivity to certain forms of conflict detection as well.

Another interesting avenue for exploration would be to examine the consequences of peer victimization or rejection on the development of cognitive performance on conflict detection tasks. Thus, for a child who is continually regulating the distress associated with being victimized, do these constant efforts compromise the child's ability to engage these same neural systems to successfully complete other types of school-related cognitive tasks? Moreover, does the impact that victimization has on cognitive abilities change as a function of developmental status, perhaps affecting younger children more than older children? Questions such as these may shed new light on developmental issues and further our understanding of the complex relationships between social and cognitive development.

Similar Psychological Processes, Different Neural Substrates

Another use for neuroimaging techniques is in determining whether distinct neural systems are involved in seemingly similar psychological processes. Showing that certain psychological processes with similar behavioral or experiential characteristics activate distinct neural regions suggests that these processes rely on separate computations and may provide insight into the ways in which these processes can be dissociated.

For example, basic behavioral research demonstrates that social estrangement can lead to emotional distress and that social connection can ameliorate these negative feelings. However, it is less clear if the negative feelings associated with social estrangement and the positive feelings associated with social connection are the product of a single system or tap into distinct underlying systems. In other words, are feelings of social estrangement and social connection two ends of the same continuum, such that feeling socially connected is the opposite of feeling socially estranged, or do these processes rely on the computations of separate underlying systems, such as has been observed with positive and negative emotions? Moreover, could there be more than one neural substrate underlying feelings of social connection, perhaps one underlying feelings of relief at not being separated and one underlying feelings of joy at being connected?

Using a parallel example from emotion research, although it was first thought that positive and negative emotion were two ends of the same spectrum, it has now been shown that positive and negative emotions rely on the computations of two dissociable systems [Cacioppo & Berntson, 1994]. This finding has led to greater specificity in understanding the ways in which these two systems can become dysregulated and how best to treat these problems. For example, it has been demonstrated that depression relates, not only to increased negative affect, but to a disturbance in the system that is implicated in positive affective experience as well [Clark & Watson,

1991]. Understanding this distinction and recognizing that certain disorders (e.g., depression) relate to altered functioning in a specific underlying system (e.g., the system that regulates positive affect) provides a more targeted way of treating specific disorders.

The extent to which feelings of social connection and feelings of social estrangement rely on common or distinct neural processes has important implications. If we assume that feelings socially connected and socially estranged rely on the same computational substrates, then the capacity to feel socially connected would be a direct correlate of one's capacity to feel socially estranged, such that those with the capacity to feel the most socially estranged would also receive the most benefit from social support. In other words, social support might only be rewarding to the extent that one is feeling socially distant. On the other hand, if feelings of social connection and social estrangement rely on the computational substrates of two separate systems, then sensitivity to social ties or a lack thereof should be dissociable, such that individuals who feel the most socially connected can also either be low or high in sensitivity to rejection or social estrangement. Moreover, this two-system approach also suggests that psychological well-being may depend not only on the absence of negative social interactions, but also on the presence of positive social interactions.

In addition, identifying the basic neural architecture that responds to social connection and estrangement may be critical for understanding how early social ties influence later social development. For example, it has been shown that the presence of abuse during childhood leads to very different psychological outcomes than does neglect or the absence of affection. Children who have been exposed to early abuse seem to show a heightened sensitivity to negative emotional cues that signify harm or aggression (such as angry faces) [Pollak & Kistler, 2002], whereas neglected children tend to show a different psychological profile characterized by avoiding social interactions altogether or showing indiscriminate friendliness towards all [Wismer Fries & Pollak, 2004]. Part of the reason for these different behavioral profiles may be due to the fact that these early experiences shape the sensitivity of separate neural systems, and thus may have different consequences for psychological function.

Clarifying Neurocognitive Mechanisms

Neuroimaging can also be used to elucidate the types of neurocognitive mechanisms underlying complex behaviors. Because behavior is the final output of the functioning of several underlying neural systems, the causes of that behavior can be multiply determined. Neuroimaging techniques allow researchers to investigate the types of computational processes that give rise to certain psychological experiences or behaviors and can be especially useful when examining the predictors of certain behaviors that are difficult to examine with self-report or behavioral measures alone.

For example, it is difficult to determine if greater emotional reactivity among children is due to: (a) a heightened sensitivity to emotional cues and thus a more intense emotional experience, (b) a diminished capacity to successfully regulate emotional states or (c) some combination of both [Fox, 2004; Posner & Rothbart, 1998]. While these processes can be difficult to disentangle with traditional behavioral methods, they may be more easily dissociated with neuroimaging methods. If emotional reactivity is due to a greater sensitivity to negative emotional stimuli, emotionally reactive children, compared to less emotionally reactive children, should show greater activity in emotion-related neural regions (such as the dACC, insula or PAG in response to social rejection or the amygdala in response to viewing negative emotional faces). Conversely, if emotional reactivity is due, not to a greater sensitivity to emotional stimuli, but rather to poorer regulatory ability, then emotionally reactive children, compared to less emotionally reactive children, should show reduced activity in prefrontal regions like the RVPFC, typically associated with emotion-regulatory processes, in response to negative emotional stimuli [Hariri et al., 2000; Lieberman et al., 2005; Petrovic & Ingvar, 2002].

Predictors of Aggression. Similar types of distinctions can be made with regard to aggressive behavior in children. A large amount of developmental work has shown that negative social experiences early on, such as abuse or rejection, can increase an individual's risk for later behavioral problems such as aggression or antisocial behavior [Dodge & Pettit, 2003]. However, a complete understanding of how these early experiences influence later behavioral problems or what neurocognitive sensitivities are being altered has not been well specified. For example, when children act aggressively, what are the underlying neurocognitive sensitivities that lead to these specific behavioral outputs?

Researchers have identified several different subtypes of aggression-related disorders, such as conduct disorder, psychopathy and antisocial personality disorder (for comprehensive reviews on the development of aggressive behavior and psychopathy, see Dodge & Pettit [2003] and Blair, Peschardt, Budhani, Mitchell, & Pine [2006], respectively). Although all of these disorders involve antisocial or aggressive behavior as a functional outcome, the experiential predictors of this behavior can vary. For example, a core feature of psychopathy is a lack of empathy, anxiety and guilt [Frick, O'Brien, Wootton, & McBurnett, 1994]. This stands in contrast to reactive aggression, which is triggered by a negative event and is associated with greater emotional reactivity to the event [Crick & Dodge, 1996]. Thus, it has been suggested [Blair et al., 2006] that some subtypes of aggression-related behavior, such as psychopathy, may be best characterized by reduced reactivity in emotion-related neural regions (e.g., amygdala [Birbaumer et al., 2005]), whereas other subtypes of aggression-related behavior, such as those related to reactive aggression, may be best characterized by either enhanced reactivity of emotion-related neural regions (e.g., amygdala [Meyer-Lindenberg et al., 2006]) or by reduced activity of prefrontal regions involved in inhibiting emotional responses (e.g., orbital and ventrolateral prefrontal cortex [Anderson, Bechara, Damasio, Tranel, & Damasio, 1999; Grafman, Schwab, Warden, Pridgen, & Brown, 1996]). These experiential predictors of aggressive behavior may be differentiated using neuroimaging techniques.

As an example of this strategy, we have recently completed a study investigating the neurocognitive mediators underlying a well-established connection between a genetic polymorphism and aggressive behavior. Recent research has suggested that a functional polymorphism in the monoamine oxidase A (MAOA) gene is associated with aggressive or antisocial behavior, especially among those individuals with early adverse experience [Caspi et al., 2002]. Individuals with the low expression version of the MAOA allele ($MAOA_{LE}$), who were exposed to early adversity, were more likely to have committed violent crimes. However, while there seems to be a relationship between MAOA and aggressive behavior [Brunner, Nelen, Breakefield, Ropers, & van Oost, 1993], it is not clear how this genetic polymorphism predisposes individuals to aggression. For example, it is not clear if the $MAOA_{LE}$ is related to aggression through reduced emotional reactivity, more characteristic of psychopathy, or through increased emotional reactivity or reduced inhibitory control, more characteristic of reactive aggression.

To examine the neurocognitive mechanisms associated with this genetic profile, we investigated how different allelic variants of the MAOA gene related to neural responses to social rejection [Eisenberger, Way, Taylor, Welch, & Lieberman, in press]. If $MAOA_{LE}$ is related to aggressive behavior through reduced emotional reactivity or reduced social concern, then $MAOA_{LE}$ individuals should show reduced dACC reactivity to social rejection as they presumably care less about social relationships or being socially included. This reduced social concern may then lead to aggressive behavior because these individuals care less about harming others or the consequences of doing so. If, however, $MAOA_{LE}$ is related to aggressive behavior through a heightened sensitivity to negative emotional experiences like social rejection, then $MAOA_{LE}$ individuals should show greater dACC activity and/or reduced RVPFC activity to social rejection as these individuals should be hypersensitive to these types of negative social experiences and unable to regulate these responses. This heightened sensitivity to negative social experiences may then result in defensively aggressive behavior (e.g., reactive aggression). Indeed, a large literature has shown that being rejected can trigger aggressive responses [Dodge & Pettit, 2003; Dodge et al., 2003; Twenge, 2005].

Results indicated that $MAOA_{LE}$ individuals, compared to those with the high expression allele ($MAOA_{HE}$), showed higher levels of self-reported trait aggression as well as greater dACC activity to social rejection [Eisenberger et al., 2006], suggesting that the relationship between this genetic polymorphism and aggressive behavior may be due to heightened, rather than reduced, emotional reactivity to negative social cues like rejection. The MAOA polymorphism was not associated with RVPFC activity or other regulatory-related prefrontal activity, suggesting that the MAOA gene may be more closely tied to emotional reactivity than to regulatory capacity. In addition, dACC reactivity to social rejection mediated the relationship between the MAOA gene and trait aggression.

Thus, it is possible that the MAOA polymorphism is related to a heightened sensitivity to negative social cues and that aggressive behavior is the functional output of this heightened sensitivity, rather than the direct consequence of this polymorphism. Obviously, future studies will need to include a measure of aggressive behavior to more clearly investigate whether individuals with the low expression allele who show greater dACC activity to social rejection are also more likely to show aggressive tendencies following rejection episodes. However, this study provides a first step in understanding the neurocognitive and experiential correlates of specific genetic profiles and thus how these genetic profiles may contribute to behavioral outcomes, like aggression. Showing that this aggressive behavior is due to heightened social sensitivity rather than reduced social sensitivity has important implications for the types of interventions that could be developed to treat these aggressive problems.

As illustrated here, one additional use of neuroimaging techniques is in elucidating the neurocognitive mechanisms that mediate genetic contributions to affect, behavior and cognition [Hariri & Weinberger, 2003]. This area may be of particular interest to developmental psychologists as a great deal of work has now shown that early social experiences can impact the expression of certain genes, thus contributing to different neurocognitive reactivities and thus to different behavioral outcomes

[Caspi et al., 2002; Fox et al., 2005]. Exploring gene-by-environment interactions may be a powerful way to understand which individuals are most likely to be negatively affected by early negative social experiences and which individuals may be spared.

Conclusion

Although research examining the neural substrates of different types of social experiences is expanding at an increasingly rapid rate, we still have much to learn. Developmental psychologists are needed in this endeavor to help elucidate how these social and emotional skills develop and the ways in which these processes can go awry. The present review has attempted to briefly outline some of the neural structures involved in the painful experience associated with broken social bonds and then to suggest some of the ways in which neuroimaging techniques can be useful in investigating how these neural systems mature, how they interact with other neural systems and how early experience may shape their development.

While some developmental questions have been posed here (e.g., what are the consequences of the same neural structures being involved in both social pain and conflict detection processes?), there are many more questions that can be asked and hopefully answered. For example, do the patterns of neural activation to social rejection look the same in children as they do in adults? Do children have more difficulty regulating the negative feelings associated with socially painful experience, and does this make the experience more distressing? Are there gender differences in neural responses to social pain? If so, are they altered as a function of puberty?

It is important that the growing amount of research on the neural correlates of adult social experience is balanced by research exploring the development of these same psychological processes in children. Through interdisciplinary research that examines psychological development at different levels of analysis, we may be able to better understand the critical impact that social ties have on normal human development. Techniques such as neuroimaging may provide new ways of understanding the developing social brain.

Acknowledgements

I would like to thank Matthew D. Lieberman and two anonymous reviewers for providing valuable feedback and suggestions on this paper. I would also like to thank Elisheva F. Gross for guiding me through some of the developmental literature and for encouraging me to think carefully about the neural correlates of social development. This work was supported by a postdoctoral research fellowship from the National Institutes of Mental Health (T32 MH-019925).

References

Adolphs, R. (2003). Cognitive neuroscience of human social behaviour. *Nature Reviews Neuroscience, 4,* 165–178.

Amaral, D.G. (2003). The amygdala, social behavior, and danger detection. *Annals of the New York Academy of Sciences, 1000,* 337–347.

Anderson, S.W., Bechara, A., Damasio, H., Tranel, D., & Damasio, A.R. (1999). Impairment of social and moral behavior related to early damage in human prefrontal cortex. *Nature Neuroscience, 2,* 1032–1037.

Aziz, Q., Schnitzler, A., & Enck, P. (2000). Functional neuroimaging of visceral sensation. *Journal of Clinical Neurophysiology, 17,* 604–612.

Bandler, R., & Shipley, M.T. (1994). Columnar organization in the midbrain periaqueductal gray: Modules for emotional expression? *Trends in Neurosciences, 17,* 379–389.

Barch, D.M., Braver, T.S., Akbudak, E., Conturo, T., Ollinger, J., & Snyder, A. (2001). Anterior cingulate cortex and response conflict: Effects of response modality and processing domain. *Cerebral Cortex, 11,* 837–848.

Birbaumer, N., Veit, R., Lotze, M., Erb, M., Harmann, C., Grodd, W., & Flor, H. (2005). Deficient fear conditioning in psychopathy: A functional magnetic resonance imaging study. *Archives of General Psychiatry, 62,* 799–805.

Blair, R.J.R., Peschardt, K.S., Budhani, S., Mitchell, D.G.V., & Pine, D.S. (2006). The development of psychopathy. *Journal of Child Psychology and Psychiatry, 47,* 262–275.

Blakemore, S.J., Winston, J., & Frith, U. (2004). Social cognitive neuroscience: Where are we heading. *Trends in Cognitive Sciences, 8,* 216–222.

Botvinick, M.M., Braver, T.S., Barch, D.M., Carter, C.S., & Cohen, J.D. (2001). Conflict monitoring and cognitive control. *Psychological Review, 108,* 624–652.

Botvinick, M.M., Cohen, J.D., & Carter, C.S. (2004). Conflict monitoring and anterior cingulate cortex: An update. *Trends in Cognitive Sciences, 8,* 539–546.

Bowlby, J. (1969). *Attachment and loss, Vol. I: Attachment.* New York: Basic Books.

Braun, K., Lange, E., Metzger, M., & Poeggel, G. (2000). Maternal separation followed by early social deprivation affects the development of monoaminergic fiber systems in the medial prefrontal cortex of *Octodon degu. Neuroscience, 95,* 309–318.

Braun, K., & Poeggel, G. (2001). Recognition of mother's voice evokes metabolic activation in the medial prefrontal cortex and lateral thalamus of *Octodon degu* pups. *Letter to Neuroscience, 103,* 861–864.

Braver, T.S., Barch, D.M., Gray, J.R., Molfese, D.L., & Snyder, A. (2001). Anterior cingulate cortex and response conflict: Effects of frequency, inhibition and errors. *Cerebral Cortex, 11,* 825–836.

Brothers, L. (1990). The neural basis of primate social communication. *Motivation and Emotion, 14,* 81–91.

Brunner, H.G., Nelen, M., Breakefield, X.O., Ropers, H.H., & van Oost, B.A. (1993). Abnormal behavior associated with a point mutation in the structural gene for monoamine oxidase A. *Science, 262,* 578–580.

Bush, G., Luu, P., & Posner, M.I. (2000). Cognitive and emotional influences in anterior cingulate cortex. *Trends in Cognitive Sciences, 4,* 215–222.

Cacioppo, J.T. & Bernston, G.G. (1994). Relationship between attitudes and evaluative space: A critical review, with emphasis on the separability of positive and negative substrates. *Psychological Bulletin, 115,* 401–423.

Carter, C.S., MacDonald, A.W., Botvinick, M.M., Ross, L.L., Stenger, V.A., Noll, D., & Cohen, J.D. (2000). Parsing executive processes: Strategic vs. evaluative functions of the anterior cingulate cortex. *Proceedings of the National Academy of Sciences, 97,* 1944–1948.

Casey, B.J., Trainor, R., Giedd, J., Vauss, Y., Vaituzis, C.K., Hamburger, S., Kozuch, P., & Rapoport, J.L. (1997). The role of the anterior cingulate in automatic and controlled processes: A developmental neuroanatomical study. *Developmental Psychobiology, 30,* 61–69.

Caspi, A., McClay, J., Moffitt, T.E., Mill, J., Martin, J., Craig, I.W., Taylor, A., & Poulton, R. (2002). Role of genotype in the cycle of violence in maltreated children. *Science, 297,* 851–854.

Cechetto, D.F., & Saper, C.B. (1987). Evidence for a viscerotopic sensory representation in the cortex and thalamus in the rat. *Journal of Comparative Neurology, 262,* 27–45.

Ciechanowski, P., Sullivan, M., Jensen, M., Romano, J., & Summers, H. (2003). The relationship of attachment style to depression, catastrophizing and health care utilization in patients with chronic pain. *Pain, 104,* 627–637.

Clark, L.A., & Watson, D. (1991). Tripartite model of anxiety and depression: Psychometric evidence and taxonomic implications. *Journal of Abnormal Psychology, 100,* 316–336.

Crick, N.R., & Dodge, K.A. (1996). Social information-processing mechanisms in reactive and proactive aggression. *Child Development, 67,* 993–1002.

Davies, P.L., Segalowitz, S.J., & Gavin, W.J. (2004). Development of error-monitoring event-related potentials in adolescents. *Annals of the New York Academy of Sciences, 1021,* 324–328.
Davis, D.A., Luecken, L., & Zautra, A.J. (2005). Are reports of childhood abuse related to the experience of chronic pain in adulthood? A meta-analytic review of the literature. *Clinical Journal of Pain, 21,* 398–405.
Deacon, T.W. (1997). *The symbolic species: The co-evolution of language and the brain.* New York: Norton & Co.
Depue, R.A., & Morrone-Strupinsky, J.V. (2005). A neurobehavioral model of affiliative bonding: Implications for conceptualizing a human trait of affiliation. *Behavioral Brain Sciences, 28,* 313–350.
Dodge, K.A., Lansford, J.E., Salzer Burks, V., Bates, J.E., Pettit, G.S., Fontaine, R., & Price, J.M. (2003). Peer rejection and social information-processing factors in the development of aggressive behavior problems in children. *Child Development, 74,* 374–393.
Dodge, K.A., & Pettit, G.S. (2003). A biopsychosocial model of the development of chronic conduct problems in adolescence. *Developmental Psychology, 39,* 349–371.
Dollard, J., & Miller, N.E. (1950). *Personality and psychotherapy* (p. 133). New York: McGraw-Hill.
Dunckley, P., Wise, R.G., Fairhurst, M., Hobden, P., Aziz, Q., Chang, L., & Tracey, I. (2005). A comparison of visceral and somatic pain processing in the human brainstem using functional magnetic resonance imaging. *Journal of Neuroscience, 10,* 7333–7341.
Eisenberger, N.I., Gable, S.L., & Lieberman, M.D. (2006). fMRI responses relate to differences in real-world social experience. *Manuscript under review.*
Eisenberger, N.I., Jarcho, J.M., Lieberman, M.D., & Naliboff, B. (in press). An experimental study of shared sensitivity to physical pain and social rejection. *Pain.*
Eisenberger, N.I., & Lieberman, M.D. (2004). Why rejection hurts: A common neural alarm system for physical and social pain. *Trends in Cognitive Sciences, 8,* 294–300.
Eisenberger, N.I., & Lieberman, M.D. (2006). What did I do wrong? Similar neural responses to social rejection and errors. *Manuscript in preparation.*
Eisenberger, N.I., Lieberman, M.D., & Williams, K.D. (2003). Does rejection hurt: An fMRI study of social exclusion. *Science, 302,* 290–292.
Eisenberger, N.I., Way, B., Taylor, S.E., Welch, W.T., & Lieberman, M.D. (in press). Genetic variation in the *MAOA* gene predicts anterior cingulate responses to social rejection. *Biological Psychology.*
Foltz, E.L, & White, L.E. (1968). The role of rostral cingulotomy in 'pain' relief. *International Journal of Neurology, 6,* 353–373.
Fox, N.A. (2004). Temperament and early social experience form social behavior. *Annals of the New York Academy of Sciences, 1038,* 171–178.
Fox, N.A., Nichols, K.E., Henderson, H.A., Rubin, K., Schmidt, L., Hamer, D., Ernst, M., & Pine, D.S. (2005). Evidence for a gene-environment interaction in predicting behavioral inhibition in middle childhood. *Psychological Science, 16,* 921–926.
Fox, A.S., Oakes, T.R., Shelton, S.E., Converse, A.K., Davidson, R.J., & Kalin, N.H. (2005). Calling for help is independently modulated by brain systems underlying goal-directed behavior and threat perception. *Proceedings of the National Academy of Sciences, 102,* 4176–4179.
Frick, P.J., O'Brien, B.S., Wootton, J.M., & McBurnett, K. (1994). Psychopathy and conduct problems in children. *Journal of Abnormal Psychology, 103,* 700–707.
Gillath, O., Bunge, S.A., Shaver, P.R., Wendelken, C., & Mikulincer, M. (2005). Attachment-style differences in the ability to suppress negative thoughts: Exploring the neural correlates. *Neuroimage, 28,* 835–847.
Grafman, J., Schwab, K., Warden, D., Pridgen, B.S., & Brown, H.R. (1996). Frontal lobe injuries, violence, and aggression: A report of the Vietnam head injury study. *Neurology, 46,* 1231–1238.
Gundel, H., O'Connor, M.F., Littrell, L., Fort, C., & Lane, R.D. (2003). Functional neuroanatomy of grief: An fMRI study. *American Journal of Psychiatry, 160,* 1946–1953.
Hajcak, G., Holroyd, C.B., Moser, J.S., & Simons, R.F. (2005). Brain potentials associated with expected and unexpected good and bad outcomes. *Psychophysiology, 42,* 161–170.
Hajcak, G., Moser, J.S., Yeung, N., & Simons, R.F. (2005). On the ERN and significance of errors. *Psychophysiology, 42,* 151–160.
Hariri, A.R., Bookheimer, S.Y., & Mazziotta, J.C. (2000). Modulating emotional responses: Effects of a neocortical network on the limbic system. *Neuroreport, 11,* 43–48.
Hariri, A.R., & Weinberger, D.R. (2003). Imaging genomics. *British Medical Bulletin, 65,* 259–270.
Harlow, H.F. (1958). The nature of love. *American Psychologist, 13,* 673–685.
Harlow, H.F., Harlow, M.K., & Suomi, S.J. (1971). From thought to therapy: Lessons from a primate laboratory. *American Scientist, 59,* 538–549.
Harlow, H.F., & Zimmermann, R.R. (1959). Affectional responses in the infant monkey. *Science, 130,* 421–432.

Holroyd, C.B., Dien, J., & Coles, M.G.H. (1998). Error-related scalp potentials elicited by hand and foot movements: Evidence for an output-independent error-processing system in humans. *Neuroscience Letters, 242,* 65–68.
Inui, T., Tanaka, S., Okada, T., Nishizawa, S., Katayama, M., & Konishi, J. (2000). Neural substrates for depth perception of the Necker cube; a functional magnetic resonance imaging study in human subjects. *Neuroscience Letters, 282,* 145–158.
Jurgens, U., & Ploog, D.W. (1970). Cerebral representation of vocalization in the squirrel monkey. *Experimental Brain Research, 10,* 532–554.
Kalin, N.H., & Shelton, S.E. (1998). Ontogeny and stability of separation and threat-induced defensive behaviors in rhesus monkeys during the first year of life. *American Journal of Primatology, 44,* 125–135.
Kalin, N.H., Shelton, S.E., & Barksdale, C.M. (1988). Opiate modulation of separation-induced distress in non-human primates. *Brain Research, 440,* 285–292.
Kirzinger, A., & Jurgens, U. (1982). Cortical lesion effects and vocalization in the squirrel monkey. *Brain Research, 233,* 299–315.
Kosslyn, S.M. (1999). If neuroimaging is the answer, what is the question? *Philosophical Transactions of the Royal Society of London, 354,* 1283–1294.
Ladouceur, C.D., Dahl, R.E., & Carter, C.S. (2004). ERP correlates of action monitoring in adolescence. *Annals of the New York Academy of Sciences, 1021,* 329–336.
Lane, R.D., Reiman, E.M., Ahern, G.L., Schwartz, G.E., & Davidson, R.J. (1997). Neuroanatomical correlates of happiness, sadness, and disgust. *American Journal of Psychiatry, 154,* 926–933.
Lieberman, M.D. (in press). Social cognitive neuroscience: A review of core processes. *Annual Review of Psychology.*
Lieberman, M.D., Gaunt, R., Gilbert, D.T., & Trope, Y. (2002). Reflection and reflexion: A social cognitive neuroscience approach to attributional inference. In M. Zanna (Ed.), *Advances in experimental social psychology* (Vol. 34, pp. 199–249). New York: Academic Press.
Lieberman, M.D., Hariri, A., Jarcho, J.M., Eisenberger, N.I., & Bookheimer, S.Y. (2005). An fMRI investigation of the associative and perceptual nature of race-related amygdala activity. *Nature Neuroscience, 8,* 720–722.
Lonstein, J.S., & Stern, J.M. (1998). Site and behavioral specificity of periaqueductal gray lesions on postpartum sexual, maternal, and aggressive behaviors in rats. *Brain Research, 804,* 21–35.
Lorberbaum, J.P., Newman, J.D., Dubno, J.R., Horwitz, A.R., Nahas, Z., Teneback, C.C., et al. (1999). Feasibility of using fMRI to study mothers responding to infant cries. *Depression and Anxiety, 10,* 99–104.
Lorberbaum, J.P., Newman, J.D., Horwitz, A.R., Dubno, J.R., Lydiard, R.B., Hamner, M.B., et al. (2002). A potential role for thalamocingulate circuitry in human maternal behavior. *Biological Psychiatry, 51,* 431–445.
MacDonald, A.W., Cohen, J.D., Stenger, V.A., & Carter, C.S. (2000). Dissociating the role of the dorsolateral prefrontal and anterior cingulate cortex in cognitive control. *Science, 288,* 1835–1838.
MacDonald, G., & Leary, M.R. (2005). Why does social exclusion hurt? The relationship between social and physical pain. *Psychological Bulletin, 131,* 202–223.
MacLean, P.D. (1985a). Brain evolution relating to family, play, and the separation call. *Archives of General Psychiatry, 42,* 405–417.
MacLean, P.D. (1985b). Evolutionary psychiatry and the triune brain. *Psychological Medicine, 15,* 219–221.
MacLean, P.D. (1993). Perspectives on cingulate cortex in the limbic system. In B.A. Vogt & M. Gabriel (Eds.), *Neurobiology of cingulate cortex and limbic thalamus: A comprehensive handbook.* Boston: Birkhauser.
MacLean, P.D., & Newman, J.D. (1988). Role of midline frontolimbic cortex in production of the isolation call of squirrel monkeys. *Brain Research, 45,* 111–123.
MacLeod, C.M., & MacDonald, P.A. (2000). Interdimensional interference in the Stroop effect: Uncovering the cognitive and neural anatomy of attention. *Trends in Cognitive Sciences, 4,* 383–391.
McEwen, B.S. (2000). The neurobiology of stress: From serendipity to clinical relevance. *Brain Research, 886,* 172–189.
Meyer-Lindenberg, A., Buckholtz, J.W., Kolachana, B., Hariri, A.R., Pezawas, L., Blasi, G., et al. (in press). Neural mechanisms of genetic risk for impulsivity and violence in humans. *Proceedings of the National Academy of Sciences.*
Mussen, P.H., & Conger, J.J. (1956). *Child development and personality* (pp. 137–138). New York: Harper.
Najib, A., Lorberbaum, J.P., Kose, S., Bohning, D.E., & George, M.S. (2004). Regional brain activity in women grieving a romantic relationship breakup. *American Journal of Psychiatry, 161,* 2245–2256.

Nelson, E.E., & Panksepp, J. (1998). Brain substrates of infant-mother attachment: Contributions of opioids, oxytocin, and norepinephrine. *Neuroscience and Biobehavioral Reviews, 22,* 437–452.
Nishina, A., Juvonen, J., & Witkow, M.R. (2005). Sticks and stones may break my bones, but names will make me feel sick: The psychosocial, somatic, and scholastic consequences of peer harassment. *Journal of Clinical Child and Adolescent Psychology, 34,* 37–48.
Ochsner, K.N. (2004). Current directions in social cognitive neuroscience. *Current Opinions in Neurobiology, 14,* 254–258.
Panksepp, J. (1998). *Affective neuroscience.* New York: Oxford University Press.
Panksepp, J., Herman, B., Conner, R., Bishop, P., & Scott, J.P. (1978). The biology of social attachments: Opiates alleviate separation distress. *Biological Psychiatry, 13,* 607–618.
Petrovic, P., & Ingvar, M. (2002). Imaging cognitive modulation of pain processing. *Pain, 95,* 1–5.
Peyron, R., Laurent, B., & Garcia-Larrea, L. (2000). Functional imaging of brain responses to pain. A review and meta-analysis. *Neurophysiological Clinics, 30,* 263–288.
Phan, K.L., Wager, T.D., Taylor, S.F., & Liberzon, I. (2004). Functional neuroimaging studies of human emotions. *CNS Spectrum, 9,* 258–266.
Phillips, M.L., Young, A.W., Senior, C., Brammer, M., Andrew, C., Calder, A.J., et al. (1997). A specific neural substrate for perceiving facial expressions of disgust. *Nature, 389,* 495–498.
Ploghaus, A., Tracey, I., Gati, J.S., Clare, S., Menon, R.S., Matthews, P.M., et al. (1999). Dissociating pain from its anticipation in the human brain. *Science, 284,* 1979–1981.
Ploog, D. (1981). Neurobiology of primate audio-vocal behavior. *Brain Research, 3,* 35–61.
Pollak, S.D. (2005). Early adversity and mechanisms of plasticity: Integrating affective neuroscience with developmental approaches to psychopathology. *Development and Psychopathology, 17,* 735–752.
Pollak, S.D., & Kistler, D.J. (2002). Early experience is associated with the development of categorical representations for facial expressions of emotion. *Proceedings of the National Academy of Sciences, 99,* 9072–9076.
Posner, M.I., & Rothbart, M.K. (1998). Attention, self-regulation, and consciousness. *Philosophical Transactions of the Royal Society of London, 353,* 1915–1927.
Quirk, G.J., Likhtik, E., Pelletier, J.G., & Pare, D. (2003). Stimulation of medial prefrontal cortex decreases the responsiveness of central amygdala output neurons. *Journal of Neuroscience, 23,* 8800–8807.
Rainville, P., Duncan, G.H., Price, D.D., Carrier, B., & Bushnell, M.D. (1997). Pain affect encoded in human anterior cingulate but not somatosensory cortex. *Science, 277,* 968–971.
Repetti, R.L., Taylor, S.E., & Seeman, T.E. (2002). Risky families: Family social environments and the mental and physical health of offspring. *Psychological Bulletin, 128,* 330–366.
Santesso, D.L., Segalowitz, S.J., & Schmidt, L.A. (2005). ERP correlates of error monitoring in 10-year-olds are related to socialization. *Biological Psychology, 70,* 79–87.
Sawamoto, N., Honda, M., Okada, T., Hanakawa, T., Kanda, M., Fukuyama, H., et al. (2000). Expectation of pain enhances responses to nonpainful somatosensory stimulation in the anterior cingulate cortex and parietal operculum/posterior insula: An event-related functional magnetic resonance imaging study. *Journal of Neuroscience, 20,* 7438–7445.
Schore, A.N. (2000). Attachment and the regulation of the right brain. *Attachment & Human Development, 2,* 23–47.
Seifritz, E., Esposito, F., Neuhoff, J.G., Luthi, A., Mustovic, H., Dammann, G., et al. (2003). Differential sex-independent amygdala response to infant crying and laughing in parents versus nonparents. *Biological Psychiatry, 54,* 1367–1375.
Smith, W. (1945). The functional significance of the rostral cingular cortex as revealed by its responses to electrical excitation. *Journal of Neurophysiology, 8,* 241–255.
Stamm, J.S. (1955). The function of the medial cerebral cortex in maternal behavior of rats. *Journal of Comparative Physiological Psychology, 47,* 21–27.
Twenge, J.M. (2005). When does social rejection lead to aggression? The influences of situations, narcissism, emotion, and replenishing connections. In K.D. Williams, J.P. Forgas & W. von Hippel (Eds.), *The social outcast: Ostracism, social exclusion, rejection, and bullying* (pp 201–212). New York: Cambridge University Press.
Williams, K., Chambers, M., Logan, S., & Robinson, D. (1996). Associations of common health symptoms with bullying in primary school children. *British Medical Journal, 313,* 17–19.
Williams, K.D., Cheung, C.K.T., & Choi, W. (2000). Cyberostracism: Effects of being ignored over the Internet. *Journal of Personality & Social Psychology, 79,* 748–762.
Wismer Fries, A.B., & Pollak, S.D. (2004). Emotion understanding in postinstitutionalized Eastern European children. *Development and Psychopathology, 16,* 355–369.
Ziabreva, I., Schnabel, R., Poeggel, G., & Braun, K. (2003). Mother's voice 'buffers' separation-induced receptor changes in the prefrontal cortex of *Octodon degu*. *Neuroscience, 119,* 433–441.

Paper

Human Development 2006;49:294–309
DOI: 10.1159/000095581

Human Development

The Discipline of Neurobehavioral Development: The Emerging Interface of Processes That Build Circuits and Skills

Elizabeth A.D. Hammock Pat Levitt

Vanderbilt University, Nashville, Tenn., USA

Key Words

Brain development · Critical period · Epigenetics · Neural circuits · Social behavior

Abstract

The study of neurobehavioral development focuses on the mechanisms through which the experiences of an individual influence the ontogeny of brain circuits that ultimately control complex functions, such as social engagement, mood and emotional regulation and cognition. Advances in experimental approaches and technologies provide opportunities to gather more detailed information about developing behavioral systems. This information is more comprehensive and readily applied in studies utilizing strategies that link the disciplines of developmental neurobiology and psychology. Here, examples are provided to illustrate the hierarchical assembly of neural systems, which incorporate information from the genome and the environment to define the ultimate developmental trajectory of an individual. Copyright © 2006 S. Karger AG, Basel

The development of all organisms is controlled by inherited traits that are encoded in the genome, and by the environment in which an individual is raised. The debate over which is more important is over, as the disciplines of biology and psychology recognize that both genes and environment are powerful forces, working together in an integrated fashion to influence all cells and organ systems. The parallels of mechanisms at work across species are, in fact, quite remarkable, allowing for direct collaboration between basic scientists and clinicians. The challenges facing neuroscientists and psychologists who study human development are two-fold: (1) defining the vulnerabilities or opportunities established developmentally through the genetic blueprint and (2) determining the mechanisms through which life experiences direct development. The central nervous system lies at the convergence of these research efforts, as it serves as the organ through which information is inter-

KARGER

Fax +41 61 306 12 34
E-Mail karger@karger.ch
www.karger.com

© 2006 S. Karger AG, Basel

Accessible online at:
www.karger.com/hde

Pat Levitt, Vanderbilt Kennedy Center for Research on Human Development
PO Box 40, Nashville, TN 37203 (USA)
Tel. +1 615 322 8242, Fax +1 615 322 5910
E-Mail pat.levitt@vanderbilt.edu

preted and synthesized for cognition and behavior. The last 30 years in neuroscience have seen an explosion of information, but the reality is that we understand precious little about the *detailed* mechanisms through which brain architecture is built, and how molecular and cellular processes are translated into complex cognitive and behavioral characteristics. Yet, it is difficult to argue that the interdisciplinary strengths of psychology and neuroscience would not benefit from a basic understanding of each other's most fundamental concepts. This paper focuses on providing examples from developmental neurobiology research that may be relevant, from a mechanistic perspective, for linking the emergence of brain circuits, reflected in an organized architecture, and the appearance of complex cognitive and behavioral functions. The discipline of *neurobehavioral development* emphasizes that development of behavioral skills begins with the gene-directed building of a biological system, which is then molded and tuned by life experience.

Why Are Genes Important, but Not Definitive?

Genetic information provides the plan for assembling cells, tissues and complex organ systems. Moreover, genes inherited from our parents not only determine key features of these systems that will in turn define the effects of experience, but can also modulate the quantity and quality of experience, by influencing the perception of experience or the motivation to attend to one particular stimulus over another. While the complete absence of a gene can result in altered neurobehavioral development, individual variation within a particular gene can also influence the way in which experience shapes neurobehavioral development. For example, in a longitudinal study in a birth cohort of 1,037 infants, variation in the monoamine oxidase A *(MAOA)* gene was found to moderate the risk of early maltreatment on anti-social behavior in adulthood [Caspi et al., 2002]. The *MAOA* gene encodes an enzyme protein that controls the levels of the neurotransmitter serotonin, which has been implicated in mood disorders and aggressive behavior. This gene is located on the X-chromosome, so males only have a single copy. While early maltreatment was associated with antisocial behavior, boys who carried the low-activity *MAOA* form of the gene were more susceptible to the effects of early maltreatment. Boys in this group, with both an environmental and genetic risk factor, made up 12% of the study cohort, but they accounted for 44% of the cohort's convictions for violent crimes. This landmark study appealed to neurobiology and psychology and was symbolic of the end of the nature-versus-nurture debate in understanding human behavior.

We know a lot about the early mechanisms that guide the formation of the brain. Developmental neurobiologists have defined the genes involved in establishing the brain plan, for example placing the cerebral cortex anterior and the brainstem posterior [Marin & Rubenstein, 2003; Rubenstein, Shimamura, Martinez, & Puelles, 1998; Wilson & Rubenstein, 2000]. Many genes and proteins that are responsible for controlling the number of neurons that are produced in any particular brain region are now known, as are the proteins that serve as guides to the nerve fibers (axons) that interconnect these regions.

A neural scaffold is established prenatally in all mammalian species [Levitt, 2003]. While the output of the genetic mechanisms can be influenced greatly by the uterine environment of the embryo and fetus (e.g., malnutrition, maternal stress, exposure to toxins or drugs of abuse), information from the outside world (experience) that stimulates patterned electrophysiological activity does not appear necessary for establishing the initial architecture of sensory and motor systems (although spontaneous prenatal brain activity does contribute to the appropriate wiring of circuits). In contrast, the work necessary after birth to build the complex systems that can interpret information and guide complex behavior depends greatly on experience. Therefore, neurobehavioral development is hierarchical: complex circuits and advanced skills depend greatly upon the capacity of earlier developing components.

The genetically influenced limits of the early developing parts of a system greatly influence the range of the subsequent developmental trajectory, and eventually the functional level and degree of plasticity the system exhibits [Knudsen, 2004]. There is an interesting mechanistic example from the hypertension literature illustrating the importance of early, genetically-guided development on later outcomes [Keller, Zimmer, Mall, Ritz, & Amann, 2003]. The number of kidney filtration units, termed glomeruli or nephrons, is predetermined by a genetic mechanism prior to birth and individuals exhibit widely different numbers of glomeruli. These glomeruli are essential for filtering body waste and regulating homeostasis by controlling the concentration of salt and other ions. How does the genetically determined number of glomeruli affect kidney function? Essentially, fewer glomeruli have to work harder to filter a specific volume of fluid in order to be as effective as a larger number of glomeruli. Individuals who died of hypertension in middle age had approximately half the number of glomeruli compared to normotensive individuals. Moreover, each glomerulus from the hypertensive individuals was almost twice the size compared to normal subjects, suggesting that over the lifetime of the individual, the glomerulus tried to adapt structurally to compensate for fewer filtration units. Here, genes guided an important aspect of kidney architecture (glomerulus number) that greatly influenced the ability to manage and adapt to lifelong environmental influences, here defined as an individual's diet. Over time, the adaptation is not sufficient to sustain normal function, perhaps because of the sheer energy drain required to maintain such an extraordinarily large filtration structure. The implication is that this failure eventually leads to dysfunction of the system. We know, however, that lifestyle can greatly affect health outcomes. Thus, it would seem possible to modify disease outcome, even in the face of altered kidney architecture, by changing the life experiences of an individual early, before the onset of hypertension, through diet and exercise. Imagine the possibilities of applying developmental psychology principles to influence positively the early developmental organization of circuits that are ultimately responsible for complex behavior. For example, it makes sense to target especially those infants who may be more likely to be in abusive situations and genetically at risk, such as the very population analyzed in the data of Caspi et al. [2002] described above, perhaps enriching the number of positive associative learning experiences for an individual.

Experience-Dependent Development

The brain is designed to efficiently process information from our environment, through primary sensory systems, and utilize these data to define appropriate responses. As mentioned above, the building of sensory systems occurs very early during fetal development. For example, by mid-gestation in primates [Kostovic, Judas, Rados, & Hrabac, 2002; Levitt, 2003; Rakic, 1977], the connections are formed from the retina, which initially processes visual information, to the thalamus, which sorts the information from both eyes. Finally, the projections reach the visual neocortex, which is responsible for integrating vast amounts of complex data and bringing it together with information from other sensory systems (e.g., we hear our name called and orient towards its origin to see who spoke it). Before that complex information processing can take place however, information from the two eyes comes together to activate neurons in the next part of the circuit. The use of both eyes during the experience-expectant 'sensitive' period of development (i.e., when the circuit is most open to change) provides the necessary patterned neurophysiological activity to modify the circuit architecture in order for the system to distinguish information coming from a particular part of their environment (visual space). Eventually, the circuit emerges as the neural representation of a precise map of visual space. But how similar is the map between individuals and what influences the quality of how well the circuit functions? A large number of recent studies have demonstrated a key role for neurons that reside locally within the circuits of the neocortex, the γ-aminobutyric acid (GABA) *interneuron* [Hensch, 2004]. The GABAergic interneuron is inhibitory in nature, essentially designed to filter and control both the information coming into a circuit, and the precision with which a circuit sends information to other brain regions. Remarkably, the interneuron is outnumbered by the larger, excitatory neurons that project long distances to other areas of the cortex that subserve different functions, or subcortically to other brain regions. In fact, the ratio of excitatory to inhibitory neurons in the adult neocortex is approximately 5:1 [Markram et al., 2004]. This ratio is conserved across all mammalian species. Moreover, the relative organization of excitatory and inhibitory neurons in the smallest functional cortical unit, the radial *minicolumn*, is identical from rodents to humans [Mountcastle, 1997; Mountcastle & Powell, 2003]. The increased capacity to mediate more complex functions in primates has its developmental origins in producing more neurons during early fetal development. The almost 1,000-fold increase in cortical surface area between mouse and human is not due to a substantial increase in cortical thickness. Rather, principles of columnar organization are maintained in the face of expansion of the neocortex by addition of minicolumns along the tangential domain [Levitt, 2003; Rakic, 1999].

Activation of circuits through experience has a potent effect on GABA neuron plasticity during development. This, in turn, defines the precision with which cortical circuits eventually mature. For example, in the visual cortex, modulation of GABA neurotransmission during the experience-expectant sensitive period, during which binocularity emerges determines the size and precision of ocular dominance columns [Fagiolini et al., 2004; Hensch et al., 1998; Hensch & Stryker, 2004]. The final outcome of this influence is relatively permanent once the maturation process is complete. That is, whatever the form of the emergent architecture, further *typical* experience will not induce additional changes. This essentially marks the closure of what is termed the *critical period*, where activity no longer influences circuit development. There is not a permanent closure of the so-called window of opportunity for imparting change in the visual system, as one can use extraordinary means to impart change in adults experimentally [Pizzorusso et al., 2002]. It is far more efficient, however, to influence the neurobiological components that mediate complex behavior early, during the experience-expectant period of development, rather than later, when systems are focused on the difficult chores of complex information processing and maintaining a healthy homeostatic balance [Knudsen, Heckman, Cameron, & Shonkoff, 2006]. We suggest that the investigations of questions pertinent to neurobehavioral development will benefit from embracing the concept that experience-dependent tuning of neural connections is a general mechanism of all brain circuits [Knudsen, 2004]. Thus, developmental concepts can be applied with equivalent rigor and meaning to complex behaviors, such as social behavior and cognition, as has occurred with primary sensory modalities.

Impacting the Neurobehavioral Hierarchy: 3 Examples

Experience Changes Developmental Timing

The handling of rodent pups during the neonatal period, or the natural variation in the care of pups by their rearing mother, can profoundly influence the developing circuits that will later control the response of an individual to environmental stressors. Manipulating the environment of the pup experimentally, by removing the neonates from the dam for a period of time each day, is also effective in changing the long-term stress response system. The biochemical and behavioral correlates have been well studied, but are there effects on the assembly of the circuit hierarchy? We have recently applied novel circuit-tracing technology that enables the investigator to determine when multisynaptic circuits are wired during development and how experience may alter the timing of circuit development [Card, Levitt, & Rinaman, 2005; Rinaman, Levitt, & Card, 2000]. The use of a reagent that contains a pseudorabies virus provides a tool for monitoring the passage of the virus across developing synapses, from one neuron in the circuit to the next in line. Thus, injecting the virus in one location results in the virus being picked up by fibers and synapses of the 'first-order' neurons, which are defined as those neurons that project directly into the area of injection. The virus, however, is only transported beyond first-order neurons to those with which they interconnect ('second'- and 'third'-order neurons). The movement from first- to second- to third-order neurons in the circuit occurs across synapses. This technology, therefore, allows one to view the timing and the qualitative nature of the labeling patterns of neurons as they become interconnected over time [Rinaman et al., 2000]. We used the organization of the brain circuits that influence autonomic functions to demonstrate this. Injection of the virus into the stomach of an animal at birth labeled the motor neurons of the vagus nerve situated in the brainstem. This shows that the nerves of the motor neurons had already reached the stomach by birth. Moreover, the virus passed backwards, across the synapses coming from neurons situated in the paraventricular nucleus of the hypothalamus, showing that the connection between the hypothalamus to the brainstem was already present by birth (fig. 1, solid arrows). No other neurons in the forebrain were labeled, even though the amygdala, cortex and other key areas that regulate stress and autonomic function send projections to the brainstem by birth (but do not yet make functional synapses). Injection of the virus 4 days later resulted in labeling of the hypothalamus again, but now the amygdala had come 'on-line'. By waiting an additional 4 days, labeling was evident in neurons situated in the cerebral cortex.

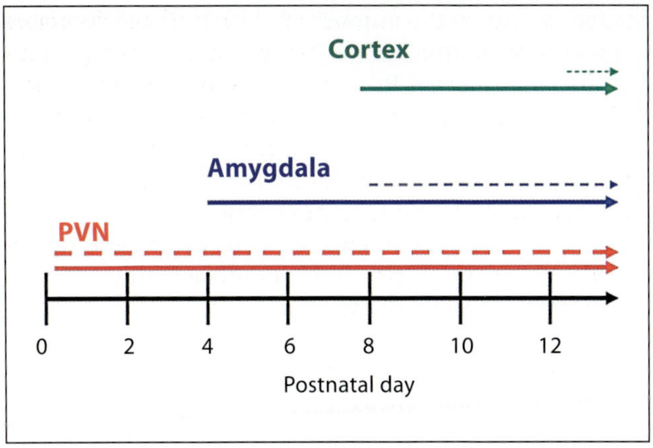

Fig. 1. Diagram summarizing the findings from pseudorabies virus studies that determined the timing of the development of autonomic circuits. The solid lines depict the period in normal animals when the labeling was achieved in the paraventricular nucleus (PVN) of the hypothalamus (red), the central nucleus of the amygdala (blue) and the cerebral cortex (green) following injection of the virus into the stomach. Labeling of neurons in these brain regions can occur only by passage of the virus across at least two synapses. The dashed lines depict the extent (thickness) and timing of neuronal labeling following brief separation of pups from their mother. The labeling in the cortex was virtually nonexistent during the first 2 weeks postnatally. The long-term outcome on final circuit formation is being investigated.

This paradigm illustrates a key aspect of neurobehavioral development, suggesting that the architecture of circuit wiring is built over time in a hierarchical fashion, from the most basic circuits that control internal physiological states (e.g., hypothalamobrainstem), to the most complex (amygdalo- or corticobrainstem) that control higher cognitive processes. Moreover, early experience can alter the timing of synapse formation that completes the wiring of the autonomic circuit. Recently, we have shown that disrupting maternal infant care for brief periods of time is sufficient to delay the formation of connections between the amygdala, cortex and the brainstem, but had little effect on the earlier developing circuit between the hypothalamus and vagal region (fig. 1, dashed arrows) [Card et al., 2005]. Thus, the timing of an experience/insult is a major determinant in defining how a particular developmental component of the circuit hierarchy will be influenced.

Experience Shapes the Biology of Stress Responses

Meaney and colleagues have published a large series of papers to show that variation in rat maternal care, especially in the quantity of pup licking and grooming, affects the neurobehavioral trajectory of the offspring. Specifically, offspring that were licked and groomed the most showed a greater ability to manage their corticosterone stress response as adults [Champagne, Francis, Mar, & Meaney, 2003; Meaney, 2001]. This can be attributed in part to the number of glucocorticoid receptors (GRs) that ultimately are expressed by neurons in the hippocampus, a brain structure well known for its role in spatial memory. GRs in the hippocampus serve as part of the long negative feedback loop from the periphery to control the activity of brain circuits that cause the release of adrenal hormones in a stress response. Thus, the stimulation of hippocampal GRs shortens the duration of the stress response. As adults, pups from mothers that provided a lower degree of licking and grooming express fewer GRs in the hippocampus. Predictably, these animals exhibit less tightly regulated, longer-duration stress responses. Cross-fostering demonstrates the remarkable power of the environment, as, in these experiments, the outcome of the stress phenotype is defined by the behavior of the mother, and not a genetic predisposition of the pup. The female offspring from the foster experience carry this phenotypic trait of stress response and maternal care forward, defining the behavior of the next generation. Recently, knowledge of the critical period for the influence of the early experience on long-term stress responsiveness, and an understanding of the developmental neurobiology led investigators to determine how the type of maternal care could influence the levels of expression of the gene encoding the GR so dramatically. The difference in experience mediated by distinct repertoires of maternal care is sufficient to change the presence of a single methyl group located on part of the GR gene that controls the level of expression, a remarkable demonstration of epigenetic 'programming', in which nonheritable factors have profound effects on the biobehavioral read-out of an individual genome [Weaver et al., 2004]. The influence of the finding is illustrated by addressing the next logical question: 'Can the stress response behavior be reversed by simply changing the methyl status of the GR gene?' In fact, administration of the amino acid L-methionine, the major precursor of the main methyl donor for DNA methylation, into the ventricles of the adult brain was sufficient to change the levels of expression of GR, stress responsiveness and the behavior of the next generation of offspring [Weaver et al., 2005]. These findings in rat models may shed light on human neonatal development. Studies in human infants and toddlers show that early life events (stress, maternal depression) can shape the way in which the child responds to adverse, stressful situations later in life [Ashman, Dawson, Panagiotides, Yamada, & Wilkins, 2002; Dawson & Ashman, 2000; Gunnar & Donzella, 2002; Jones, Field, & Fox, 1997], although the molecular mechanisms have not yet been determined.

Learning Shapes Neurobehavioral Development

In addition to the long-term effects of licking and grooming rates on stress regulation, neonatal licking and grooming appears to be an important unconditioned stimulus in early associative learning processes. Regina Sullivan and colleagues developed a model system to study olfactory learning of a socially relevant behavior [Sullivan & Leon, 1986; Sullivan, Wilson, & Leon, 1989]. In the paradigm, juvenile rats prefer a nonsocial odor, like lemon, if the odor was paired with vigorous somatosensory stimulation as neonates [Wilson, Sullivan, & Leon, 1987]. If trained in this paradigm as a neonate, juveniles spend more time with the lemon odor than with another novel odor. No such behavioral preference is observed if the odor was presented in the absence of vigorous somatosensory stimuli. Pups only learn this association when the training paradigm includes training sometime between postnatal days 1 and 8, after which the critical period closes [Woo & Leon, 1987]. In fact, even an odor paired with a normally aversive stimulus, such as a foot shock, is equally potent in driving an associative learning process during the critical period. Even with the foot shock, the neonates still exhibit a preference for the paired odor [Roth & Sullivan, 2001]. However, after the critical period, this pairing results in an aversive response to the odor. This timing coincides with the termination of the 'stress hyporesponsive' period for rats, and thus, one possibility for manipulating the system would be to change the exposure of the pups to stress hormones during the critical period. In fact, Moriceau, Wilson, Levine and Sullivan [2006] demonstrated that corticosterone-depleted animals (adrenalectomized) or animals in which GR activation is inhibited directly in the amygdala, a brain structure involved in anxiety, fear and stress responses, still showed preference for the odor when paired with the foot shock after the critical period. Thus, the timing of the dynamic change in responsiveness to the paired nonsocial odor, from attractive to aversive, is regulated specifically by the actions of the stress hormone corticosterone in developing brain circuits that are highly sensitive to experience. This model system is particularly exciting, because one can integrate well-demonstrated psychological processes, such as associative learning, with the ability to perform cross-species analyses using the same associative learning paradigm, even in human infants [Sullivan et al., 1991].

Investigating the Development of Social Behavior

Building from these three examples in the animal literature, the study of social behavior, as complex as it is, serves as an excellent example of emerging principles that guide studies of neurobehavioral development. The past 20 years of research in the neurosciences have provided irrefutable evidence that gene-environment interactions during development underlie the establishment of circuits that mediate sensory, emotional and social behaviors. Social behavior is both highly complex and diverse across animal species, exhibiting remarkable variability even within a single species. The complexity of learning specific skills that ultimately are required for typical social behavior is reflected in the remarkably extended period of time over which both the relevant brain regions (frontal and temporal lobes) and the behaviors develop in humans [Durston & Casey, 2006; Shaw et al., 2006; Webb, Monk, & Nelson, 2001]. The heterogeneity of social behavior in humans is substantial, ranging from socially reclusive to outgoing. Neurodevelopmental disorders, such as William's syndrome and autism spectrum disorders and even many neuropsychiatric disorders, such as schizophrenia, typically reside at the extremes of this continuum. As in the general population, there is substantial heterogeneity exhibited by individuals within the same disorder. Such heterogeneity could arise by qualitative or quantitative variation among individuals in their genes and neural circuits. However, heterogeneity will also be influenced greatly by experience-expectant processes underlying the development of social competence. In this regard, the factors that underlie the ontogeny of primary sensory systems are well understood, but for functions as complex as social behavior, neurobehavioral development is still very early in the discovery process. In this context, it may help to have a theoretical and research framework to investigate the mechanisms of experience-dependent ontogeny of social behavior and the sources of heterogeneity in the typical population, and in developmental disorders, such as autism.

Developmental Hierarchies and the Emergence of Social Behavior

Our model of the ontogeny of social behavior unites data from research on the molecular neurobiology of adult social behavior and the molecular and neurophysiological data from the development of sensory systems. In the model, the proper development of species-appropriate social behavioral repertoires requires a prolonged hierarchical process involving the formation and maturation of both long-distance connections and local circuits driven in part by experience-expectant learning processes, just like in primary sensory systems [Knudsen, 2004]. Thus, social formation that occurs during postnatal brain development (fig. 2) can be modeled as a gradual process where neural circuits supporting more basic functions develop first, and more sophisticated social competence emerges later as long-distance circuits are integrated (y-axis) and local circuits are finely tuned (x-axis). Internal physiological states (e.g., hunger, thirst, malaise, arousal) drive motivational processes to orient and/or move toward innately salient environmental stimuli (e.g., nipple odorants, faces, movement). At the first level, the basic neural circuitry underlying these processes is in place from birth. For example, the pseudorabies virus experiments (fig. 1) showed that the connectedness of a structure like the paraventricular nucleus in the hypothalamus, which regulates neuroendocrine aspects of homeostasis, is not modulated significantly by postnatal experience. These early homeostatic mechanisms alter motivation, which modulates attention, the antecedent to cognitive mechanisms that allow the developing neonate to begin to discriminate social versus nonsocial stimuli. This process builds to more complex social cognitive skills. The studies of Sullivan and Meaney probe the transitions for learning to discriminate and attend to more socially meaningful information at the advanced levels of the hierarchy. In humans, with the ability to detect conspecifics, infants need to discriminate among them. A more advanced level of social discrimination is the ability to discern and interpret various social signals arising from the same individual in various contexts. With further maturation, the socially competent human brain can infer complex social meaning from limited sensory stimuli and can utilize social information to optimize social encounters. Higher levels in the system cultivate feedback mechanisms to regulate lower levels in the hierarchy. In the protracted socioemotional development of humans, this prolonged development of reliable feedback mechanisms is evident in the emotional volatility of youth. Dahl [2004] and colleagues, for example, have discussed the complex changes in brain and behavior that occur during puberty, particularly related to social behavior. Disturbances in social engagement and motivation at this very complex transitional time period appear to influence adult vulnerability for anxiety and depression [Dahl, 2004; Williamson, Forbes, Dahl, & Ryan, 2005].

This model may have important implications for the observed social heterogeneity found in the general population, as well as that expressed by individuals affected by neurodevelopmental disorders, such as autism (for a review, see Pelphrey, Adolphs, & Morris [2004]). The processes underlying social competence are not all-or-none; they exist as quantitative traits. For example, an early disruption in the

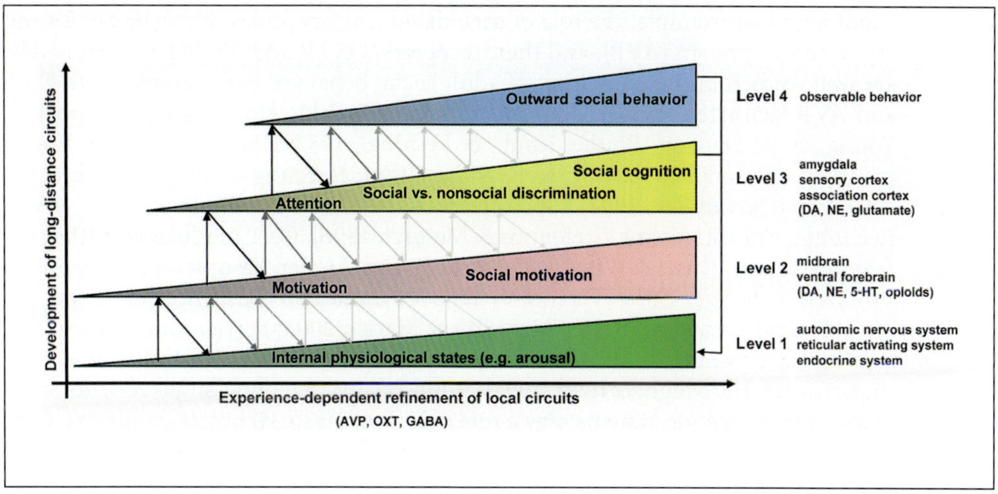

Fig. 2. A hierarchical model of the ontogeny of social behavior. The green triangle represents the earliest developing circuits, in place from birth, that control the internal physiological states that subserve motivational processes, represented in more complex circuits that are also present at birth (pink triangle). Attention to stimuli in the environment is subserved by those circuits higher in the hierarchy (yellow triangle) that provide the infant with the ability to learn how to discriminate social versus nonsocial stimuli. This builds towards more complex social cognitive skills over time. In the context of the ontogeny of social behavior, the most advanced level of social discrimination is the ability to 'read' different social signals that originate from the same individual in various contexts. Maturation of these social skills occurs through childhood, over a very long period of time, providing opportunities to gain expertise in deciphering complex social meaning from limited information, to be able to optimize social encounters. Feedback to each level of the circuit modulates both social cognitive performance and internal physiological states. Specific neural circuits, such as those that utilize the neuropeptides arginine vasopressin (AVP) and oxytocin (OXT), may interact with GABAergic systems to refine the circuitry at each level of the hierarchy. Other neuromodulators (e.g. norepinephrine, NE, and dopamine, DA) and neurotransmitters (glutamate) are also influential in mediating the formation of the hierarchy during the development of more complex social skills. 5-HT = Serotonin.

level of competence for social discrimination might alter the further development and maturation of higher-order social cognition. This would also impact the development and maturation of important feedback on internal state regulation and motivational processes. Additionally, because there are multiple circuits that comprise the developing system, qualitatively different insults could also result in atypical social behavior.

Putting the 'Neuro' into Social Behavioral Development

The hierarchical model incorporates particular circuits and systems that are likely to be involved in the ontogeny of social behavior, though there are few studies that have focused on understanding the neurobehavioral mechanisms that underlie the development of this complex behavior. There are, however, likely neurobiological candidates. For example, the role of the related neuropeptides oxytocin (OXT) and arginine vasopressin (AVP), and their receptors, OXTR and AVPR1A, respectively, are well studied in the regulation of adult social behavior. For example, both OXT and AVP facilitate social recognition behavior [Bielsky, Hu, Szegda, Westphal, & Young, 2004; Dantzer, Bluthe, Koob, & Le Moal, 1987; Dluzen, Muraoka, Engelmann, & Landgraf, 1998; Ferguson, Aldag, Insel, & Young, 2001; Kendrick et al., 1997; Popik & Van Ree, 1992; Popik, Vetulani, & Van Ree, 1992; Popik, Vos, & Van Ree, 1992; van Wimersma Greidanus & Maigret, 1996]. OXT modulates mother-infant interactions [Insel & Winslow, 1991; Pedersen, Ascher, Monroe, & Prange, 1982; Pedersen & Prange, 1979; Winslow et al., 2000], and AVP influences male species-typical social behaviors [Bester-Meredith & Marler, 2003; Ferris, Albers, Wesolowski, Goldman, & Luman, 1984; Goodson, Lindberg, & Johnson, 2004; Winslow, Hastings, Carter, Harbaugh, & Insel, 1993]. Additionally, in monogamous rodents, both of these neuropeptide systems play a role in long-term social bonds [Williams, Carter, & Insel, 1992; Winslow et al., 1993; Young & Wang, 2004]. Individual and species differences in brain OXTR density in a region of the brain, which mediates rewarding behavior, correlate with a propensity to engage spontaneously in nurturing behavior in several rodent species [Olazabal & Young, 2006a, 2006b]. Furthermore, genetic variation in *avpr1a* predicts variation in receptor distribution patterns and social heterogeneity in adult male prairie voles [Hammock & Young, 2005]. It is important to emphasize, however, that in contrast to extensive information in the adult, there is relatively little known regarding OXT and AVP systems during the ontogeny of social behavior.

There are several reasons supporting a hypothesis for both neuropeptides playing central roles during development. First, OXT, AVP and their receptors are expressed at different levels and in unique patterns during fetal and postnatal development [Buijs, Velis, & Swaab, 1980; Wang, Liu, Young, & Insel, 1997; Wang & Young, 1997; Wang, Young, Liu, & Insel, 1997]. Second, separation-induced vocalizations are reduced in neonatal mice with genetic disruption of OXT [Winslow et al., 2000] or OXTR [Takayanagi et al., 2005], and are also reduced in neonatal rats given a central infusion of OXT [Insel & Winslow, 1991]. Third, neonatal manipulation of either system alters adult behavior in the prairie vole [Bales & Carter, 2003]. Fourth, treatment of neonatal voles with an OXTR antagonist increases aggression directed toward infants when the treated animals are later tested as juveniles [Bales, Kim, Lewis-Reese, & Carter, 2004]. Fifth, 7 days of treatment with AVP in neonates increases aggression in adult male prairie voles [Stribley & Carter, 1999]. Sixth, the Brattleboro rat, which has a genetic mutation that prevents the proper production of AVP, exhibits altered brain development [Boer, Van Rheenen-Verberg, & Uylings, 1982], including effects on neurotransmitter content [Boer, Feenstra, Botterblom, Korse, & Te Riele, 1995; Scholer & Sladek, 1982]. Additionally, as adults, the Brattleboro rat has deficits in social recognition behavior [Engelmann & Landgraf, 1994] and in prepulse inhibition of startle [Feifel & Priebe, 2001], both of which are disrupted in autism spectrum disorders. Although less is known about the roles of these neuropeptides in human social behavior, several reports have implicated dysregulation of OXT and AVP systems in autism [Green et al., 2001; Hollander et al., 2003; Kim et al., 2002; Modahl et al., 1998; Wassink et al., 2004; Wu et al., 2005] and in the modulation of human social behavior by OXT and AVP in typical adults [Kosfeld, Heinrichs, Zak, Fischbacher, & Fehr, 2005; Thompson, George, Walton, Orr, & Benson, 2006].

The investigation of social behavior ontogeny may thus be best achieved using neurobehavioral development principles. For example, given the role of GABA in the experience-dependent development of sensory circuits, and the well-established roles of OXT and AVP in social behavior, it makes sense from a neurobiological perspective to determine the relative interactions between these signaling pathways in influencing the development of the 'social brain'.

Conceptualizing Studies of Social Learning and Experience-Expectant Development

Model systems that cross species boundaries are particularly attractive for deciphering the neurobehavioral basis for the emergent properties of a functional system. This can be done for the ontogeny of social behavior, incorporating principles of hierarchical neurobehavioral development and using the neonatal olfactory learning paradigm described by Sullivan and colleagues as mentioned above. Thus, for neonatal rodents, social valence may be assigned to maternally provided somatosensory stimulation (e.g. licking and grooming) during a period of heightened learning in an experience-dependent fashion. Licking and grooming is among the first postnatal sensory stimuli, as are the odors of the nest and surrounding conspecifics. Social valence may be acquired through an experience-expectant associative learning process. This process begins as enhanced circuit activity, perhaps of OXT and AVP systems, which during licking and grooming may define the coincident neural representation of the surrounding nest and conspecifics as 'social'. Such associative learning then allows other stimuli to become conditioned and acquire social properties through nth-order associative learning mechanisms. The convergent activity of circuits would facilitate the development of important feedback circuitry to regulate OXT and AVP systems more precisely. In our own studies, we have suggested that local GABAergic interneurons may play this role of local tuning in key 'social' forebrain and cortical areas, just as it has been determined for primary sensory systems. Predicted from this model is that feedback would result in the release of OXT and AVP in olfactory and forebrain regions in future social contexts, without the need for licking and grooming. Later in development, exposure to other sensory modalities with the social odor alone would generate OXT and AVP release. As animals become more mobile and mature, the simultaneous activity of several sensory modalities labeled as 'social' may begin to fine-tune the cortex to allow for control of species-appropriate social behavior. This general model of the ontogeny of social behavior is currently being tested in mouse studies.

Neurobehavioral Development as an Aspiring Discipline

The cross-disciplinary efforts in brain and behavior are no longer considered exceptional. Cognitive neuroscience utilizes the power of monitoring brain activation patterns in real time, during task performance, to define the circuit correlates of typical and atypical functioning. In the context of cognitive skill development, structural imaging is now revealing that the trajectory of brain growth may be more important than the absolute size the cerebral cortex achieves [Shaw et al., 2006].

Thus, knowledge of the course of development, and the particular experiences and environments to which one is exposed, is essential for understanding outcomes in both typical and atypical populations. Moreover, the integration of research disciplines has led to the recent discovery of a correlation between having certain variations in the sequences of genes encoding proteins involved in neural circuit function, such as catechol-O-methyltransferase, and the quality of cognitive performance [Egan et al., 2001; Tunbridge, Harrison, & Weinberger, 2006]. There is increasing speculation that such genetic variants create a more or less vulnerable substrate for disordered thinking, such as in schizophrenia. Developmentally, vulnerability to pathological environments may be determined in part by variations in which form of the serotonin transporter one inherits [Caspi et al., 2003]. Thus, the neurobiology of the early developing systems and circuits, established through genetic mechanisms, provides the basis for, and may define, the qualitative and quantitative nature of how any individual integrates experiences into their behavioral repertoire that may last a lifetime. The parallels with other nonneural functions, such as structure-function relationships in hypertension, are uncanny. The study, therefore, of child development, from a well-integrated biobehavioral perspective, seems both logical and essential.

Acknowledgements

We thank Dr. Kathie Eagleson for helpful comments regarding the manuscript and Drs. Peter Mundy, Wendy Stone, Paul Yoder and Daniel Messinger for discussions of the social hierarchy model as part of the Vanderbilt-Miami Marino Autism Research Institute. Effort of the authors was supported in part by NIMH MH67842 (to P.L.), NICHD Core Grant P30 HD15052 to the Vanderbilt Kennedy Center (to P.L.) and NIH Roadmap Training Grant T32 MH075883 (to E.A.D.H.).

References

Ashman, S.B., Dawson, G., Panagiotides, H., Yamada, E., & Wilkins, C.W. (2002). Stress hormone levels of children of depressed mothers. *Development and Psychopathology, 14,* 333–349.

Bales, K.L., & Carter, C.S. (2003). Developmental exposure to oxytocin facilitates partner preferences in male prairie voles *(Microtus ochrogaster). Behavorial Neuroscience, 117,* 854–859.

Bales, K.L., Kim, A.J., Lewis-Reese, A.D., & Carter, C.S. (2004). Both oxytocin and vasopressin may influence alloparental behavior in male prairie voles. *Hormonal Behavior, 45,* 354–361.

Bester-Meredith, J.K., & Marler, C.A. (2003). Vasopressin and the transmission of paternal behavior across generations in mated, cross-fostered *Peromyscus* mice. *Behavioral Neuroscience, 117,* 455–463.

Bielsky, I.F., Hu, S.B., Szegda, K.L., Westphal, H., & Young, L.J. (2004). Profound impairment in social recognition and reduction in anxiety-like behavior in vasopressin V1a receptor knockout mice. *Neuropsychopharmacology, 29,* 483–493.

Boer, G.J., Feenstra, M.G., Botterblom, M.J., Korse, V., & Te Riele, P. (1995). Early postnatal appearance of enhanced noradrenaline content in the brain of vasopressin-deficient Brattleboro rat: Normal adrenoceptor densities and aberrant influences of vasopressin treatment. *International Journal of Developmental Neuroscience, 13,* 63–74.

Boer, G.J., Van Rheenen-Verberg, C.M., & Uylings, H.B. (1982). Impaired brain development of the diabetes insipidus Brattleboro rat. *Brain Research, 255,* 557–575.

Buijs, R.M., Velis, D.N., & Swaab, D.F. (1980). Ontogeny of vasopressin and oxytocin in the fetal rat: Early vasopressinergic innervation of the fetal brain. *Peptides, 1,* 315–324.

Card, J.P., Levitt, P., & Rinaman, L. (2005). Early experience modifies the postnatal assembly of autonomic emotional circuits in the rat. *Journal of Neuroscience, 25,* 9102–9111.

Caspi, A., McClay, J., Moffitt, T.E., Mill, J., Martin, J., Craig, I.W., et al. (2002). Role of genotype in the cycle of violence in maltreated children. *Science, 297,* 851–854.
Caspi, A., Sugden, K., Moffitt, T.E., Taylor, A., Craig, I.W., Harrington, H., et al. (2003). Influence of life stress on depression: Moderation by a polymorphism in the 5-HTT gene. *Science, 301,* 386–389.
Champagne, F.A., Francis, D.D., Mar, A., & Meaney, M.J. (2003). Variations in maternal care in the rat as a mediating influence for the effects of environment on development. *Physiological Behavior, 79,* 359–371.
Dahl, R.E. (2004). Adolescent brain development: A period of vulnerabilities and opportunities – Keynote address. *Annals of the New York Academy of Sciences, 1021,* 1–22.
Dantzer, R., Bluthe, R.M., Koob, G.F., & Le Moal, M. (1987). Modulation of social memory in male rats by neurohypophyseal peptides. *Psychopharmacology, 91,* 363–368.
Dawson, G., & Ashman, S.B. (2000). *On the origins of a vulnerability to depression: The influence of the early social environment on the development of psychobiological systems related to risk for affective disorder.* Mahwah, N.J.: Erlbaum & Assoc.
Dluzen, D.E., Muraoka, S., Engelmann, M., & Landgraf, R. (1998). The effects of infusion of arginine vasopressin, oxytocin, or their antagonists into the olfactory bulb upon social recognition responses in male rats. *Peptides, 19,* 999–1005.
Durston, S., & Casey, B.J. (2006). What have we learned about cognitive development from neuroimaging? *Neuropsychologia, 44,* 2149–2157.
Egan, M.F., Goldberg, T.E., Kolachana, B.S., Callicott, J.H., Mazzanti, C.M., Straub, R.E., et al. (2001). Effect of COMT Val108/158 Met genotype on frontal lobe function and risk for schizophrenia. *Proceedings of the National Academy of Sciences of the United States of America, 98,* 6917–6922.
Engelmann, M., & Landgraf, R. (1994). Microdialysis administration of vasopressin into the septum improves social recognition in Brattleboro rats. *Physiological Behavior, 55,* 145–149.
Fagiolini, M., Fritschy, J.M., Low, K., Mohler, H., Rudolph, U., & Hensch, T.K. (2004). Specific $GABA_A$ circuits for visual cortical plasticity. *Science, 303,* 1681–1683.
Feifel, D., & Priebe, K. (2001). Vasopressin-deficient rats exhibit sensorimotor gating deficits that are reversed by subchronic haloperidol. *Biological Psychiatry, 50,* 425–433.
Ferguson, J.N., Aldag, J.M., Insel, T.R., & Young, L.J. (2001). Oxytocin in the medial amygdala is essential for social recognition in the mouse. *Journal of Neuroscience, 21,* 8278–8285.
Ferris, C.F., Albers, H.E., Wesolowski, S.M., Goldman, B.D., & Luman, S.E. (1984). Vasopressin injected into the hypothalamus triggers a stereotypic behavior in golden hamsters. *Science, 224,* 521–523.
Goodson, J.L., Lindberg, L., & Johnson, P. (2004). Effects of central vasotocin and mesotocin manipulations on social behavior in male and female zebra finches. *Hormonal Behavior, 45,* 136–143.
Green, L., Fein, D., Modahl, C., Feinstein, C., Waterhouse, L., & Morris, M. (2001). Oxytocin and autistic disorder: alterations in peptide forms. *Biological Psychiatry, 50,* 609–613.
Gunnar, M.R., & Donzella, B. (2002). Social regulation of the cortisol levels in early human development. *Psychoneuroendocrinology, 27,* 199–220.
Hammock, E.A., & Young, L.J. (2005). Microsatellite instability generates diversity in brain and sociobehavioral traits. *Science, 308,* 1630–1634.
Hensch, T.K. (2004). Critical period regulation. *Annual Review of Neuroscience, 27,* 549–579.
Hensch, T.K., Fagiolini, M., Mataga, N., Stryker, M.P., Baekkeskov, S., & Kash, S.F. (1998). Local GABA circuit control of experience-dependent plasticity in developing visual cortex. *Science, 282,* 1504–1508.
Hensch, T.K., & Stryker, M.P. (2004). Columnar architecture sculpted by GABA circuits in developing cat visual cortex. *Science, 303,* 1678–1681.
Hollander, E., Novotny, S., Hanratty, M., Yaffe, R., DeCaria, C.M., Aronowitz, B.R., et al. (2003). Oxytocin infusion reduces repetitive behaviors in adults with autistic and Asperger's disorders. *Neuropsychopharmacology, 28,* 193–198.
Insel, T.R., & Winslow, J.T. (1991). Central administration of oxytocin modulates the infant rat's response to social isolation. *European Journal of Pharmacology, 203,* 149–152.
Jones, N.A., Field, T., & Fox, N.A. (1997). EEG activation in 1-month-old infants of depressed mothers. *Development and Psychopathology, 9,* 491–505.
Keller, G., Zimmer, G., Mall, G., Ritz, E., & Amann, K. (2003). Nephron number in patients with primary hypertension. *New England Journal of Medicine, 348,* 101–108.
Kendrick, K.M., Da Costa, A.P., Broad, K.D., Ohkura, S., Guevara, R., Levy, F., et al. (1997). Neural control of maternal behaviour and olfactory recognition of offspring. *Brain Research Bulletin, 44,* 383–395.
Kim, S.J., Young, L.J., Gonen, D., Veenstra-Vander Weele, J., Courchesne, R., Courchesne, E., et al. (2002). Transmission disequilibrium testing of arginine vasopressin receptor 1A (AVPR1A) polymorphisms in autism. *Molecular Psychiatry, 7,* 503–507.

Knudsen, E., Heckman, J.J., Cameron, J.L., & Shonkoff, J.P. (2006). Economic, neurobiological, and behavioral perspectives on building America's future workforce. *Procedings of the National Academy of Sciences of the United States of America, 103,* 10155–10162.
Knudsen, E.I. (2004). Sensitive periods in the development of the brain and behavior. *Journal of Cognitive Neuroscience, 16,* 1412–1425.
Kosfeld, M., Heinrichs, M., Zak, P.J., Fischbacher, U., & Fehr, E. (2005). Oxytocin increases trust in humans. *Nature, 435,* 673–676.
Kostovic, I., Judas, M., Rados, M., & Hrabac, P. (2002). Laminar organization of the human fetal cerebrum revealed by histochemical markers and magnetic resonance imaging. *Cerebral Cortex, 12,* 536–544.
Levitt, P. (2003). Structural and functional maturation of the developing primate brain. *Journal of Pediatrics, 143,* S35–S45.
Marin, O., & Rubenstein, J.L. (2003). Cell migration in the forebrain. *Annual Review of Neuroscience, 26,* 441–483.
Markram, H., Toledo-Rodriguez, M., Wang, Y., Gupta, A., Silberberg, G., & Wu, C. (2004). Interneurons of the neocortical inhibitory system. *National Review of Neuroscience, 5,* 793–807.
Meaney, M.J. (2001). Maternal care, gene expression, and the transmission of individual differences in stress reactivity across generations. *Annual Review of Neuroscience, 24,* 1161–1192.
Modahl, C., Green, L., Fein, D., Morris, M., Waterhouse, L., Feinstein, C., et al. (1998). Plasma oxytocin levels in autistic children. *Biological Psychiatry, 43,* 270–277.
Moriceau, S., Wilson, D.A., Levine, S., & Sullivan, R.M. (2006). Dual circuitry for odor-shock conditioning during infancy: Corticosterone switches between fear and attraction via amygdala. *Journal of Neuroscience, 26,* 6737–6748.
Mountcastle, V.B. (1997). The columnar organization of the neocortex. *Brain, 120,* 701–722.
Mountcastle, V.B., & Powell, T.P. (2003). Introduction: Computation in cortical columns. *Cerebral Cortex, 13,* 2–4.
Olazabal, D.E., & Young, L.J. (2006a). Oxytocin receptors in the nucleus accumbens facilitate 'spontaneous' maternal behavior in adult female prairie voles. *Neuroscience, 141,* 559–568.
Olazabal, D.E., & Young, L.J. (2006b). Species and individual differences in juvenile female alloparental care are associated with oxytocin receptor density in the striatum and the lateral septum. *Hormonal Behavior, 49,* 681–687.
Pedersen, C.A., Ascher, J.A., Monroe, Y.L., & Prange, A.J., Jr. (1982). Oxytocin induces maternal behavior in virgin female rats. *Science, 216,* 648–650.
Pedersen, C.A., & Prange, A.J., Jr. (1979). Induction of maternal behavior in virgin rats after intracerebroventricular administration of oxytocin. *Procedings of the National Academy of Sciences of the United States of America, 76,* 6661–6665.
Pelphrey, K., Adolphs, R., & Morris, J.P. (2004). Neuroanatomical substrates of social cognition dysfunction in autism. *Mental Retardation and Developmental Disabilities Research Reviews, 10,* 259–271.
Pizzorusso, T., Medini, P., Berardi, N., Chierzi, S., Fawcett, J.W., & Maffei, L. (2002). Reactivation of ocular dominance plasticity in the adult visual cortex. *Science, 298,* 1248–1251.
Popik, P., & Van Ree, J.M. (1992). Long-term facilitation of social recognition in rats by vasopressin related peptides: A structure-activity study. *Life Science, 50,* 567–572.
Popik, P., Vetulani, J., & Van Ree, J.M. (1992). Low doses of oxytocin facilitate social recognition in rats. *Psychopharmacology, 106,* 71–74.
Popik, P., Vos, P.E., & Van Ree, J.M. (1992). Neurohypophyseal hormone receptors in the septum are implicated in social recognition in the rat. *Behavioral Pharmacology, 3,* 351–358.
Rakic, P. (1977). Prenatal development of the visual system in the rhesus monkey. *Biological Science, 278,* 245–260.
Rakic, P. (1999). Setting the stage for cognition: Genesis of the primate cerebral cortex. In M.S. Gazzaniga (Ed.), *The New Cognitive Neurosciences* (2nd ed., pp. 7–21). Cambridge: MIT Press.
Rinaman, L., Levitt, P., & Card, J.P. (2000). Progressive postnatal assembly of limbic-autonomic circuits revealed by central transneuronal transport of pseudorabies virus. *Journal of Neuroscience, 20,* 2731–2741.
Roth, T.L., & Sullivan, R.M. (2001). Endogenous opiates and their role in odor preference acquisition and consolidation following odor-shock conditioning in infant rats. *Developmental Psychobiology, 39,* 188–198.
Rubenstein, J.L., Shimamura, K., Martinez, S., & Puelles, L. (1998). Regionalization of the prosencephalic neural plate. *Annual Review of Neuroscience, 21,* 445–477.
Scholer, J., & Sladek, J.R., Jr. (1982). An altered noradrenergic innervation of the Brattleboro rat supraoptic nucleus. *Annals of the New York Academy of Sciences, 394,* 718–728.
Shaw, P., Greenstein, D., Lerch, J., Clasen, L., Lenroot, R., Gogtay, N., et al. (2006). Intellectual ability and cortical development in children and adolescents. *Nature, 440,* 676–679.

Stribley, J.M., & Carter, C.S. (1999). Developmental exposure to vasopressin increases aggression in adult prairie voles. *Procedings of the National Academy of Sciences of the United States of America, 96,* 12601–12604.
Sullivan, R.M., & Leon, M. (1986). Early olfactory learning induces an enhanced olfactory bulb response in young rats. *Brain Research, 392,* 278–282.
Sullivan, R.M., Taborsky-Barba, S., Mendoza, R., Itano, A., Leon, M., Cotman, C.W., et al. (1991). Olfactory classical conditioning in neonates. *Pediatrics, 87,* 511–518.
Sullivan, R.M., Wilson, D.A., & Leon, M. (1989). Norepinephrine and learning-induced plasticity in infant rat olfactory system. *Journal of Neuroscience, 9,* 3998–4006.
Takayanagi, Y., Yoshida, M., Bielsky, I.F., Ross, H.E., Kawamata, M., Onaka, T., et al. (2005). Pervasive social deficits, but normal parturition, in oxytocin receptor-deficient mice. *Procedings of the National Academy of Sciences of the United States of America, 102,* 16096–16101.
Thompson, R.R., George, K., Walton, J.C., Orr, S.P., & Benson, J. (2006). Sex-specific influences of vasopressin on human social communication. *Procedings of the National Academy of Sciences of the United States of America, 103,* 7889–7894.
Tunbridge, E.M., Harrison, P.J., & Weinberger, D.R. (2006). Catechol-O-methyltransferase, cognition, and psychosis: Val158Met and beyond. *Biological Psychiatry, 60,* 141–151.
van Wimersma Greidanus, T.B., & Maigret, C. (1996). The role of limbic vasopressin and oxytocin in social recognition. *Brain Research, 713,* 153–159.
Wang, Z., Liu, Y., Young, L.J., & Insel, T.R. (1997). Developmental changes in forebrain vasopressin receptor binding in prairie voles *(Microtus ochrogaster)* and montane voles *(Microtus montanus). Annals of the New York Academy of Sciences, 807,* 510–513.
Wang, Z., & Young, L.J. (1997). Ontogeny of oxytocin and vasopressin receptor binding in the lateral septum in prairie and montane voles. *Brain Research Developmental Brain Research, 104,* 191–195.
Wang, Z., Young, L.J., Liu, Y., & Insel, T.R. (1997). Species differences in vasopressin receptor binding are evident early in development: comparative anatomic studies in prairie and montane voles. *Journal of Comparative Neurology, 378,* 535–546.
Wassink, T.H., Piven, J., Vieland, V.J., Pietila, J., Goedken, R.J., Folstein, S.E., et al. (2004). Examination of AVPR1a as an autism susceptibility gene. *Molecular Psychiatry, 9,* 968–972.
Weaver, I.C., Cervoni, N., Champagne, F.A., D'Alessio, A.C., Sharma, S., Seckl, J.R., et al. (2004). Epigenetic programming by maternal behavior. *Nature Neuroscience, 7,* 847–854.
Weaver, I.C., Champagne, F.A., Brown, S.E., Dymov, S., Sharma, S., Meaney, M.J., et al. (2005). Reversal of maternal programming of stress response in adult offspring through methyl supplementation: Altering epigenetic marking later in life. *Journal of Neuroscience, 25,* 11045–11054.
Webb, S.J., Monk, C.S., & Nelson, C.A. (2001). Mechanisms of postnatal neurobiological development: Implications for human development. *Developmental Neuropsychology, 19,* 147–171.
Williams, J.R., Carter, C.S., & Insel, T. (1992). Partner preference development in female prairie voles is facilitated by mating or the central infusion of oxytocin. *Annals of the New York Academy of Sciences, 652,* 487–489.
Williamson, D.E., Forbes, E.E., Dahl, R.E., & Ryan, N.D. (2005). A genetic epidemiologic perspective on comorbidity of depression and anxiety. *Child and Adolescent Psychiatric Clinics of North America, 14,* 707–726.
Wilson, D.A., Sullivan, R.M., & Leon, M. (1987). Single-unit analysis of postnatal olfactory learning: Modified olfactory bulb output response patterns to learned attractive odors. *Journal of Neuroscience, 7,* 3154–3162.
Wilson, S.W., & Rubenstein, J.L. (2000). Induction and dorsoventral patterning of the telencephalon. *Neuron, 28,* 641–651.
Winslow, J.T., Hastings, N., Carter, C.S., Harbaugh, C.R., & Insel, T.R. (1993). A role for central vasopressin in pair bonding in monogamous prairie voles. *Nature, 365,* 545–548.
Winslow, J.T., Hearn, E.F., Ferguson, J., Young, L.J., Matzuk, M.M., & Insel, T.R. (2000). Infant vocalization, adult aggression, and fear behavior of an oxytocin null mutant mouse. *Hormonal Behavior, 37,* 145–155.
Woo, C.C., & Leon, M. (1987). Sensitive period for neural and behavioral response development to learned odors. *Brain Research, 433,* 309–313.
Wu, S., Jia, M., Ruan, Y., Liu, J., Guo, Y., Shuang, M., et al. (2005). Positive association of the oxytocin receptor gene (OXTR) with autism in the Chinese Han population. *Biological Psychiatry, 58,* 74–77.
Young, L.J., & Wang, Z. (2004). The neurobiology of pair bonding. *Nature Neuroscience, 7,* 1048–1054.

Commentary

Human Development 2006;49:310–314
DOI: 10.1159/000095582

Human Development

Biology's Useful Contribution: A Comment

Jerome Kagan

Harvard University, Cambridge, Mass., USA

Key Words
Behavior · Brain · Infancy

The history of every natural science affirms the seminal truth that new sources of evidence pertinent to a fruitful construct usually lead to theoretical advances. The novel information, often the product of a new technology, is accompanied either by parsing the extant idea into two or more categories, rejecting the concept or affirming its validity. For example, when physicists became capable of measuring microwave radiation from the cosmos the data forced them to posit the two new forms of matter called dark energy and dark matter. The invention of X-ray crystallography provided information allowing Crick and Watson to infer the correct structure of the gene and to reject older conceptions.

Psychology and the other social sciences have not enjoyed equally frequent introductions of new methodologies. This unfortunate state of affairs is especially frustrating to investigators who study humans and their development. Verbal statements and observed behaviors, usually in laboratory contexts, continue to be, as they have for centuries, the two primary sources of data, even though many investigators suspected that important advances would follow the ability to quantify brain activity. The excellent papers by Nelson, Moulson and Richman, Eisenberger, and Hammock and Levitt confirm this intuition.

Nelson and colleagues describe how event-related potentials and scanning technologies have clarified the concepts of a face schema and explicit, or retrieval, memory. The biological evidence implies that both competences develop gradually and

KARGER

Fax +41 61 306 12 34
E-Mail karger@karger.ch
www.karger.com

© 2006 S. Karger AG, Basel
0018–716X/06/0495–0310$23.50/0

Accessible online at:
www.karger.com/hde

Jerome Kagan
Department of Psychology, Harvard University
Cambridge, MA 02138 (USA)
Tel. +1 617 495 3870, Fax +1 617 495 3728
E-Mail jk@wjh.harvard.edu

their structures during infancy differ from the forms they assume in adults. Behavioral observations had hinted at this important fact earlier [Kagan & Herschkowitz, 2005], but the event-related potential evidence rendered this speculation a more trusted fact and, as a dividend, provided guides to others regarding the measurements they should use if they pursued these questions. I suspect that if investigators recorded event-related potentials in infants, in addition to the traditional measure of duration of attention, the observations would provoke some skepticism over the claim that infants under 1 year can 'add' and 'know' that an object cannot pass through a solid barrier.

Eisenberger, who advocates functional magnetic resonance imaging technology to elaborate behavioral and self-report evidence on complex emotional states, summarizes intriguing relations between activation of the dorsal anterior cingulate and the psychological states of rejection or exclusion. There are, however, two potential problems with her conclusions.

First, when different incentives produce the same biological reaction in a person, it is not always legitimate to infer a similar psychological state. For example, an imminent attack, memorizing a string of numbers, and exercise are all accompanied by an increase in heart rate, but no investigator would conclude that the psychological states evoked by these conditions are similar. Similarly, certain sites in the motor cortex that represent the muscles of the hand would be activated if a person picked up a stone, struck a person or caressed a lover, even though the psychological states were distinct. The amygdala is activated by photographs of snakes and erotic scenes.

A second problem derives from reliance on metaphors to persuade colleagues of a broad generalization. Although humans say that burning their hand and feeling rejected are 'painful' experiences, scientists should not apply the term 'pain' to the latter condition. The word 'bit' in the sentences 'The boy bit the apple' and 'The governor bit the bullet' do not have the same meaning because its use in the second sentence is metaphorical.

It is important to know that the dorsal anterior cingulate cortex is activated in a laboratory setting when individuals report feeling excluded from a group. However, as Eisenberger notes, other areas of the brain were activated at the same time. Hence, the dorsal anterior cingulate is only one component of a complex brain response, and it is likely that the complete profiles of activation for the experiences of physical pain and rejection are distinctive.

Hammock and Levitt remind us of the importance of timing and the brain's preparedness for select experiences. They also affirm the maxim that interactions between genetic vulnerabilities and experience, and not main effects for either, are to be expected. Hence, those who look for genetic determinants should be as careful in the environmental evidence they gather as they are in quantifying the biological information. The same imperative applies to those who gather psychological measures to quantify experience.

Although the finding by Caspi et al. [2003] is to be celebrated, readers should appreciate that the best predictor of antisocial behavior is a childhood of poverty and inadequate schooling. Epidemiological data imply that about 8 of 10 adolescents who engage in gang violence or robbery are characterized by this profile, whereas it is estimated that only 1 of 10 has the monoamine oxidase A polymorphism. And most with the polymorphism never commit an antisocial act. The celebration of material, biological causes over the nonmaterial psychological forces by Western scholars is the reason for the acclaim awarded to reports of gene-by-environment interactions. I agree with the suggestion that infants in potentially abusive homes should be removed to more benign settings or the parents persuaded to adopt nurturant regimens. Both strategies are difficult in modern democracies where family privacy is defended.

The hope that research on animals will illuminate many issues relevant to human development is especially strong among American investigators who take the Darwinian premise seriously. No one questions the fact that animal models for physiological functions have proven valuable. But psychological constructs pose a special problem because children impose a symbolic appraisal on their experience that rodents do not. There can be no animal model for the psychological state of a child from an ethnic minority who is chronically teased by peers or for an adolescent girl who has been sexually abused by her father. The neurochemical systems that have been shown to have dramatic effects on animal behavior are relevant to humans. However, these molecules establish a general state of the nervous system from which a large, though limited, number of outcomes is possible. No scientist has shown that any neurotransmitter or receptor distribution has a uniform effect on a human psychological measure. That is why adults from middle- versus lower-class backgrounds react differently to the same biological intervention and why the heritability of some of the talents measured on IQ tests are about 0.50 for middle-class children but close to zero for poor children. A mouse who fails to explore a brightly lit alley seems to share features with a shy child. But apparent similarities of this kind are too easy to infer and can be due to different mechanisms. The brain and psychological state that provoke a female rhesus monkey to mate with a half dozen males over the course of a day are different from those of a woman who engages in exactly the same behavior. I applaud the imaginative studies of animal behavior and read them with great interest. They could prove relevant to some human psychological states. But I suspect that when their relevance is discovered scholars will be surprised by the features that turned out to have significance. If Pavlov were able to read the contemporary literature on conditioning he would have to retract many of his bold claims, including the positing of a 'freedom reflex'. Nature is a compulsive architect who loves specificity in the details and apparently takes delight in informing scientists who thought they had uncovered a big secret: 'Sorry, wrong.'

Final Comments

Despite the importance of adding biological measures to behaviors and self-reports, all is not 'sweetness and light' because there is incomplete commensurability among the metrics and structures that characterize the three sources of evidence. I have argued [Kagan, 2006] that all natural phenomena consist of cascades of processes with each component in a cascade described with a distinct vocabulary. Unfortunately, it is not always possible to translate the vocabulary appropriate for the elements of one phase into the language appropriate for the succeeding phase. The semantic forms used to describe brain processes, and the inferences drawn from the information, are not appropriate for the propositions that describe beliefs, emotions and instrumental actions.

Humans, across all cultures, use the dimensions of good-bad and high-low salience when they use words or sentences to describe objects, events, people and feelings [Osgood, Suci, & Tannenbaum, 1957]. The metric for the relations among semantic terms is strength of association or semantic distance. As a result, individuals classify the emotional states called rage and terror as semantically similar because both are salient and undesired, even though the conditions that provoke them, their sensory qualities, behavioral consequences and accompanying brain profiles are different.

The metrics and structures of behaviors are less clear for there are no cross-cultural studies of the usual reactions to a number of varied incentives. However, a primary metric for behaviors is rate of change in the frequency of responses over time. I suspect that the profile of behaviors evoked by a stranger insulting a person's family would differ, in all cultures, from the profile observed when agents encountered strangers holding a dagger. Hence, behavioral data would place the concepts rage and terror in distinct categories.

Measures of brain activity, like event-related potentials in the EEG and profiles of blood flow assessed with functional magnetic resonance imaging scanners, rely on other distinctive metrics (e.g. the metric for event-related potential waveforms is a set of changes in latency and magnitude over time in particular sites). Although most scientists have not compared the brain reaction following an insult to an agent's family with the reaction to a threat of bodily harm, I suspect that these two incentives would produce distinct profiles, and the relations between them would differ from the relations noted for semantic forms and overt behaviors. As a result, each source of evidence – semantic reports, behaviors and brain activity – would lead to a different conclusion regarding the relation between rage and terror. Hurricanes can be described in terms of their potential cost in dollars, the diameter of the storm in kilometers, the velocity in kilometers per hour, and the percent of water molecules in the air mass. Each class of measure for a psychological construct has a distinct metric and structure. There may be utility in categorizing psychological states, or processes, in accord with combinations of the expectedness and familiarity of the incentive event, subsequent brain states, the cognitive processes that accompany those brain states, and, finally, in children over 2 years of age, the valence and salience of the imposed semantic interpretations. A change in any one of those features might represent a unique psychological state. The perception of color provides an analogy.

Although the 1,269 color chips in the Munsell system can be derived from combinations of the three dimensions of value, hue and chroma, humans can discriminate among all 1,269 colors [Wyszecki & Stiles, 1982]. On some occasions it is useful to treat all red surfaces as similar; on others it will be more fruitful to distinguish crimson from pink. A similar conclusion is appropriate for psychological states. Eisenberger argued that it might be fruitful to regard all instances of activation of the dorsal anterior cingulate as representing a similar emotional state, even though behavioral and self-report evidence indicates that the emotions generated by touching a hot stove and feeling rejected by friends are different.

The addition of biological information to behavioral and self-report evidence, which is to be applauded, will reveal that many current psychological constructs are far too abstract and fail to accommodate to the extraordinary specificity in nature. Measures of brain activity will force psychologists to specify, more exactly than they have, the nature of the incentive (social or nonsocial), the source of evidence (behavior, self-report, event-related potentials), the context in which the measurement occurs (laboratory, school, home), and the age, social class, gender and, on some occasions, the cultural background of the individuals being evaluated. It is time to compose conclusions with full sentences rather than the naked predicates that dominate the contemporary literature.

References

Caspi, A., McClay, J., Moffitt, T.E., Mill, J., Martin, J., Craig, I.W., et al. (2002). Role of genotype in the cycle of violence in maltreated children. *Science, 297,* 851–854.

Caspi, A., Sugden, K., Moffitt, T.E., Taylor, A., Craig, I.W., Harrington, H., McClay, J., Mill, J., Martin, J., Braithwaite, A., & Poulton, R. (2003). Influence of life stress on depression: Moderation by a polymorphism in the 5-HTT gene. *Science, 301,* 386–389.

Kagan, J. (2006). *An argument for mind.* New Haven, CT: Yale University Press.

Kagan, J., & Herschkowitz, N. (2005). *A young mind in a growing brain.* Mahwah, N.J.: Erlbaum.

Osgood, C.E., Suci, G.J., & Tannenbaum, T.H. (1957). *The measurement of meaning.* Urbana, IL: University of Illinois Press.

Wyszecki, G., & Stiles, W.S. (1982). *Color science: concepts and methods, qualitative data, and formulae* (2nd ed.). New York: Wiley.

Author Index Vol. 49, No. 5, 2006

Human Development

Subject Index Vol. 49, No. 5, 2006

© 2006 S. Karger AG, Basel

Fax +41 61 306 12 34
E-Mail karger@karger.ch
www.karger.com
Accessible online at:
www.karger.com/hde